ABORTION
Facts and
Feelings

A Handbook for
Women and the
People Who Care
About Them

ABORTION
Facts and
Feelings

A Handbook for
Women and the
People Who Care
About Them

Nada L. Stotland, M.D.

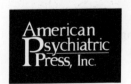

American
Psychiatric
Press, Inc.

Washington, DC
London, England

Copyright © 1998 American Psychiatric Press, Inc.
ALL RIGHTS RESERVED
Manufactured in the United States of America on acid-free paper
First Edition
01 00 99 98   4 3 2 1
American Psychiatric Press, Inc.
1400 K Street, N.W., Washington, DC   20005
www.appi.org

Library of Congress Cataloging-in-Publication Data
Stotland, Nada Logan.
    Abortion : facts and feelings : a handbook for women and the
people who care about them / Nada L. Stotland. — 1st ed.
        p.   cm.
    Includes bibliographical references and index.
    ISBN 0-88048-740-2
    1. Pregnant women—Mental health—Handbooks, manuals, etc.
2. Abortion—Psychological aspects—Handbooks, manuals, etc.
I. Title.
RG588.S86   1998
618.8′8′019—dc21   97-35435
                                                                           CIP

British Library Cataloguing in Publication Data
A CIP record is available from the British Library.

To my cherished daughters
Lea, Naomi, Eve, and Hanna
and all the women of the past, present, and future

Contents

Acknowledgments

The author extends her thanks to Anjali Bhorade, Eve Stotland, and Jennifer Jo Kim, without whose dedicated and creative research assistance this book would not have been possible.

The author also wishes to acknowledge the outstanding research and editorial contributions of Jennifer Lang Kim.

Why This Book?

Where do you turn when you are wrestling with a painful decision? You turn to trusted friends and relatives, to professionals, to religious advisers. But sometimes you want accurate information and suggestions all in one place, in a form you can use on your own.

This book is for women who are considering whether or not to have an abortion; women who have had an abortion and want to do more thinking about it; and relatives, mates, lovers, friends, and health professionals who want to help the women they care for make the best possible choices for themselves.

The decision to have an abortion is not an easy one, and it is not the right decision for every pregnant woman, even in difficult circumstances. Every situation is different. Women considering abortion range in age from 9 to 55 years. They are rich and poor; married and unmarried; white, black, brown, yellow, and red; members of every religious group and ethnic origin; heterosexual and homosexual. Some have no one to talk to and others have too many people talking to them. Some are in danger from physical, sexual, and emotional abuse.

None of us knows how our life and circumstances will develop in the future. We can never be sure how we will feel about a decision we make now, one week, one year, and many years later. We can never know how the other alternatives would have worked out.

The decision of whether to have an abortion is also made under the time pressures of pregnancy. While a woman is thinking about it, her pregnancy may progress beyond the point at which an abortion can be performed. The pregnancy will soon be visible to everyone. If a pregnancy is not terminated, a baby will be born in a few short months.

This book was written because partners in relationships, families, and friends, as well as pregnant women themselves, deserve to have accurate information about this common but controversial procedure—information they can use to make both personal and policy decisions. This book contains that information.

Author's Perspective

The statements in this book are based on a careful review of the medical and other relevant literature. This book also includes and respects a wide variety of philosophical and religious approaches to pregnancy. I feel strongly that women have the right to make their own individual, informed, and supported reproductive choices. It would be wonderful if no pregnancy were ever a problem, but in reality, that has never happened and probably never will happen. No one can ensure that any decision will be a perfect one. But when a pregnancy is a problem, no one can know better than the woman herself what she can do and what she needs to do about it. Society could and should do more to support mothers. But no one should be able to make a woman stay pregnant and become a mother, make it difficult for her to get a medically safe abortion, harass her in the process of getting an abortion, or make her risk the terror, shame, and danger of illegal abortion.

Definition

The word *abortion* is used in this book to indicate a medical or surgical procedure that is performed to end a pregnancy. (In the medical literature, the term *abortion* or *spontaneous abortion* is also used to indicate a miscarriage.)

SECTION 1

For Women . . .

CHAPTER 1

Problem Pregnancy: Approaching a Decision

You are not alone. There are approximately 1.5 million abortions performed each year in the United States.[1,2] At present rates, 46% of women will have an abortion at some time in their lives.[3,4] Women of all colors, all religions, all ages, and all walks of life have abortions. Many other statistical facts about abortion and related reproductive events will be found in the chapters that follow, but here are just a few recent facts reported by the Alan Guttmacher Institute, which conducts research on abortion, in 1995:

- More than 50% of pregnancies among U.S. women are unintended, and half of these unintended pregnancies are terminated by abortion.
- Each year nearly 3 of every 100 women ages 15–44 have abortions.

- Each year, approximately 46% of women obtaining abortions have had at least one previous abortion, and 53% have had at least one previous birth.
- Most women obtaining abortions are young; 55% are under age 25, whereas only 22% are age 30 and older.
- Pregnant unmarried women are six times more likely than married women to obtain abortions.
- Poor women are about three times more likely to have abortions than women who are not poor.
- Eleven percent of all abortions are obtained by women with a household income of $50,000 or more.
- White women account for 63% of all abortions.
- However, nonwhite women are twice as likely to have an abortion than are white women.
- The number of abortions performed for every 100 Hispanic women is 43% higher than that among every 100 non-Hispanic women.
- Catholic women are 30% more likely than Protestant women to have abortions, but women who report no religious affiliation have a higher abortion rate than women reporting some religious affiliation.
- Although "born-again" or evangelical Christians are only about half as likely as other women to obtain abortions, in 1987 one in six abortion patients described herself as a born-again or evangelical Christian.
- Seventy percent of women obtaining abortions report that they intend to have children in the future.

Approaching the Decision

The decision whether to have an abortion is always made at a time of crisis.[5] It is a crisis to have significant doubts about whether it is a good idea to continue a pregnancy. Perhaps your pregnancy was begun deliberately and happily, but since conception your circumstances have drastically changed: perhaps your partner has abruptly left or changed his mind about wanting a baby, financial support has vanished, or there is a family or vocational emergency or serious concern about your physical or emotional health. Perhaps the pregnancy was unplanned: there was no time or money to get contraceptive help, your partner objected to the use of contraception, the contraceptive method failed. You are filled with emotions. How could this happen? Where are the people I counted on? What will other people think? What is the right thing to do? How will I manage? What are my options?

Taking the decision-making process step by step will enable you to make the best possible decision for your own circumstances. Even in a time crunch, it is important to take a deep breath, stop, and review the situation from several perspectives. Following are some questions to ask yourself in order to clarify your thinking. It is surprising how often the right decision becomes clear after you have given yourself the emotional space and information you need.

Questions to Ask Yourself

✦ Your Background

What kind of attitudes about sex, pregnancy, abortion, and motherhood were you raised with?
What attitudes do you hold now?

✦ Your Religion

What are your religious beliefs and affiliations?
How does your religion view abortion, adoption, and child rearing for someone in your situation?

✦ Your Hopes and Plans

What are your wishes and plans for the immediate, midterm, and long-term future?
How much control do you feel you have over your own future?

◆ Your Personal Traits

What are the personal strengths and weaknesses you bring to the
   situation? Consider factors such as
   Your maturity
   Your intelligence
   Your education
   Your ability to nurture others
   Your ability to organize
   Your energy level

◆ How Your Decision Would Influence Your Future

How would you adapt to each of the alternatives—abortion, child
   rearing, or adoption—now and over time?

◆ What Information Do You Have? Need?

What do you know about
   Abortion
   Pregnancy
   Childbirth
   Adoption
   Caring for a child?
What are the abortion laws where you live?
Do you know where to obtain an abortion? How would you find
   out?

◆ Who Is Important and Helpful to You?

How will your decision affect people who are important to you, and
   how will their reactions affect you?
Do you want anyone to help you make your decision, and if so, who
   would it be?
Who may give you emotional and other kinds of support for whatever decision you make, or only for one or the other?

◆ What Are Your Circumstances?

Are there important financial aspects of your situation? What financial alternatives do you have?

Do you have, can you get, and can you keep a job to support yourself and a child?

Can you afford the housing you need?

◆ How Are You Doing?

Is the situation so upsetting that it is affecting your physical or emotional health or preventing you from making up your mind? Do you need professional psychological help?

Outcomes

The best outcomes result when women, in consultation with others if they wish, make and carry out the decisions they think are best, without pressure or coercion, and receive support for their decisions from the people they care about. Under these circumstances, abortion is a physically and psychologically safe choice for the vast majority of pregnant women who choose it, and the physical and psychological outcomes of abortion for the woman are as good or better than those of childbirth.[4,6–9]

Abortion in Context

Again, you are not alone. Women have faced decisions about abortion in all times and places. Abortion has been practiced since ancient times and continues to be practiced in every kind of society all over the world. This book provides information on:

- The practice of abortion in other times and places, as well as practical information about how it is practiced now
- Some of the laws that were in force while this book was being writ-

ten, and how to find out which laws apply where you live and in other places where you might go

- The attitudes of major North American religious groups about abortion and how to obtain more specific information about the approaches of your religion
- The medical and psychological outcomes of abortion
- The alternatives to abortion—delivering the baby and either caring for it yourself or allowing someone else to provide the parenting: in other words, adoption
- The needs and concerns of women in special circumstances and of women's loved ones

Most important, this book will help you think through and carry out your own decision, whatever it is. It may be read as a whole, or individual chapters may be consulted as needed.

Where Does This Information Come From?

The information and suggestions in this book come from the scientific literature and from the clinical experiences of the author, a physician who specializes in psychiatry, especially in psychological aspects of obstetrics and gynecology. A reference list is included at the back of the book.

Scientific, or medical, evidence is information that has been subjected to statistical analysis and to the review of experts in the field and that has been selected for publication in medical journals. This is in contrast to what is called "anecdotal" evidence, which consists of individuals' stories about medical treatments or procedures and their outcomes in individual cases.

Anecdotes can be emotionally powerful. One frightening or adverse outcome can convince a physician, a patient, or an observer that a medication is dangerous or a treatment is traumatic, despite the fact that many others have been treated without ill effects. In studying the impact of abortion, it is essential to remember that the circumstances of a condition or treatment have a significant impact on the outcome. The same physical wound feels very different when it is the result of war, street violence, an accident, or a sport. The experience of nausea and vomiting is very different depending on whether it results from cancer chemotherapy, pregnancy, or a gastrointestinal infection, what help is available, and what the person experiencing it thinks is going to happen to her. Information about the circumstances of medical events like abortion is crucial to scientific study of the outcome of those events.

Another requirement for scientific evidence is the use of "control subjects." These are people who resemble the patients being studied, except for the treatment being studied; control patients may have undergone a different treatment for the same condition or no treatment at all. To understand the outcomes of abortion, it is most reasonable to compare them with the outcomes of uninterrupted pregnancy, because uninterrupted pregnancy is the only available alternative to abortion.

More Definitions

This book doesn't use the traditional terms *doctor* and *patient*. Nowadays there are many professions that can be involved in the care of a pregnant woman. And a healthy woman, pregnant or not, may not think of herself as a "patient." A woman and her health care professional(s) work together, exchanging information, making decisions, and carrying out medical treatment. Good health care requires mutual trust and cooperation.

Another important definition concerns the nature of the pregnancies that may lead a woman to consider an abortion and to look for information. It may seem obvious that these pregnancies are "unwanted." However, that is not always true. They may have been started deliberately under circumstances that have now drastically changed. Pregnancies may be, and often are, "unwanted" in one sense but not in another; that is, the woman may wish to remain pregnant, but she may feel that having a baby in a few months would not be fair to her family, herself, the baby, or children she would like to have in the future. The term *unintended pregnancy* has also been used to describe these pregnancies. But, just as a pregnancy may be intended but unwanted, a pregnancy may be unintended but wanted. Many "accidental" conceptions become valued pregnancies and cherished children.

So the term *problem pregnancy* will be used in this book. It means only that the question of continuing or terminating the pregnancy presents a problem to the pregnant woman. The decision to end a pregnancy is a personal life decision that can be carried out, and is most safely carried out, by a medical intervention: an induced abortion. The word *abortion* in this book means induced abortion.

In many of the disputes about the morality and legality of abortion, the opposing sides are referred to as "pro-choice" and "pro-life." The term *pro-life* is chosen by groups that oppose the legalization of abortion. It implies that those who support legalized abortion are opposed to life itself. This is neither fair nor true. Life exists in many forms, including plant and animal, human and nonhuman.

The answer to the question of when human life begins is not simple. The fertilization of an egg by a sperm does not result in a fully formed human being. Development into a human being requires a very complicated set of conditions, including development inside the body of a woman. In addition to the potential human life represented by the pregnancy, there are the lives of the mother and others to consider. Although we would like to value and support all human life equally, no society ever has or currently is able to do so. Making safe and legal abortion unavailable exposes women to the serious risks of unsafe, illegal abortion.

Being in favor of reproductive choice, including abortion, does not mean being in favor of abortion. It means allowing each person to make whatever decision she finds necessary to her values and her situation, even when some of those decisions are painful to her or to others. "Pro-choice" respects the right of women who are against abortion for religious or other personal reasons not to have abortions. Abortion is, at best, a painful choice.

CHAPTER 2

Why Do We Feel the Way We Do About Abortion?

I t is helpful to understand abortion in the context of women's reproductive situations and choices throughout history and in other societies as well as our own. Abortion is neither a new idea nor a symbol of the breakdown of morals. Abortion has been practiced throughout history and in every known society, whether or not it was socially acceptable, legal, or physically safe.

Historical Perspectives

Abortion is described in medical manuscripts dating from ancient Greece. Abortion was known by the ancient Hebrews and is mentioned in historical documents from every era.[1]

In Western society in general, until late in the 1800s abortion was considered acceptable up to the time of "quickening," when the pregnant woman feels the movement of the fetus.[2] Women's magazines routinely carried advertisements for drugs and instruments women used (effectively or not) for abortion. Around this time, physicians organized to recognize obstetrics and gynecology as a medical specialty and to claim the care of pregnant women from the traditional midwives, who had often performed both abortions and deliveries for the women in their communities. During the Victorian era, doctors emphasized the "natural," primary role of women as wives and mothers and exerted considerable pressure on women to marry and bear children. For the first time, abortion was outlawed.

Abortion and Society

Women living in societies without modern contraceptive and abortion techniques do not always conceive and bear one child after another throughout their reproductive lives. By one means or another, births are limited. Sizes and spacings of families vary greatly, according to social custom and economic circumstances. Some societies value large families, whereas others value small ones. External attempts to impose changes in these values on a population, whether by encouraging new behaviors or discouraging or limiting traditional ones, often fail.

Anthropologists report that every known society practices some means to end pregnancies.[3] Abortion methods used in other societies include substances women take by mouth, insert into their vaginas, or rub onto their skin; the application of heat; the insertion of pointed objects into the uterus; and physical pressure on the lower abdomen.

There have been eras in both ancient and modern civilizations during which authorities launched major campaigns to convince potential parents to have several children. Nevertheless, the size of the average family continued to shrink. For example, effective contraceptive methods were largely unavailable in communist Russia. Despite an official policy encouraging larger families, shortages of housing, child care, child care necessities, and basic consumer goods made it very difficult for urban Russians to provide for more than one child. Abortion was legal and was provided, though without anesthesia, by the state health system. The average Russian woman underwent approximately nine abortions during her lifetime.[4]

In contrast, the government of China, deeply concerned about its ability to house and feed its mushrooming population, launched a campaign to induce couples to limit their families to one child. A strong Chinese cultural tradition favors male children and requires sons to carry on the family name and to care for aging parents. Hence the posters and other media messages in China encouraging one-child families feature parents with a single angelic daughter, who can now aspire to all the careers once limited to males.

Newly married couples who agree to sign pledges to have only one child are given special consideration for housing and other scarce resources. These benefits continue for them and for the first child, who is admitted to special schools and pediatric care. If the couple has a second child, however, all the special family benefits stop. There is close surveillance of married women, including public charting of their menstrual periods, to make sure that the rules for reproduction are not violated. When a woman becomes pregnant without official permission, community authorities exert intense pressure on her to terminate the pregnancy by abortion. Despite all these efforts, people living outside the major metropolitan areas, and particularly in agricultural regions where children assist in family farming, continue to have larger families than the authorities allow.

Other societies take abortion for granted. In modern-day Japan, birth control pills are not legally available. Condoms are available, but some men refuse to use them. Abortion is legal and generally socially acceptable.[1] It is also recognized that an abortion ends the possibility of a particular potential life, and that women may feel sad about the loss even as they decide that abortion is the best choice in a particular situation. Many Japanese practice the Shinto religion. The Shinto goddess dedicated to infants and small children takes an interest in aborted embryos as well. Women who have abortions may bring offerings in the form of baby bibs or toys to the shrines of this goddess in order to make peace with the souls of children they chose not to bear.

Social Attitudes Toward Women, Sex, and Reproduction: Are Women to Blame for Problem Pregnancies?

Attitudes toward abortion are related to attitudes and assumptions about the roles of women in sex and reproduction. In many societies, both past and present, the responsibility for sexual behavior is placed almost entirely on women. If an unmarried man and woman have sexual intercourse, the woman is much more likely than the man to be considered immoral, promiscuous, and unclean. Even when the woman is too young to give legal consent, is the victim of incest, or is physically or psychologically forced into the act, society often tends to question her behavior rather than that of the man who took advantage of her. How was she dressed? How did she behave? What neighborhood was she in? A woman who becomes pregnant under these circumstances may be shunned, banned, or even killed. Her pregnancy may bring shame to her family. Her prospects for marriage may be over. She may, and often does, resort to an abortion even if it is illegal, painful, and dangerous.

In North America, contraceptive methods are generally legal and available, and recent studies indicate that contraceptive use, specifically condom use, is on the rise among U.S. women.[5] However, contraceptive methods can and do fail. In fact, studies of U.S. women obtaining abortions consistently find that one-half or more of these women were practicing some method of contraception during the month in which they became pregnant.[6,7] The realities of women's lives can interfere with the effective use of contraception. Many women lack the necessary information about reproduction, feel uncomfortable about sex and contraception, or worry about the side effects of contraceptives. Many women do not feel powerful enough in their relationships to refuse sex or to insist that contraception be used. Some women cannot afford contraceptives or trips to a clinic for contraceptive advice. Some men insist on intercourse and refuse to use or allow contraception.

Nevertheless, the woman who experiences an unanticipated or unwelcome pregnancy may be considered, or may even consider herself, sexually irresponsible. This attitude adds an extra burden to the decision about how to handle the pregnancy.

Other Alternatives: Childbirth, Adoption, Unconventional Families

Attitudes toward adoption are related to views about the relationship between biological relationship and parenthood. Some societies and social groups accept mothers and children who do not conform to the usual family groupings. Social views toward the adoption of infants by family members, friends, or unrelated prospective parents vary widely. In some groups, adoption is considered a generous act of both the birth mother and the adoptive parent(s)—a decision that frees the birth mother of a responsibility she is not able to assume, offers the rewards of parenthood to an adult or couple not able to produce biological children, and gives the child a wanted place in a secure home.

In other social groups, adoption is viewed as unnatural and unacceptable:[8] for the birth mother, it is seen as a rejection of her maternal attachments and responsibilities, and for the adoptive parent(s), it is perceived as a suspicious willingness to accept a "stranger" into the intimacy of the family. Children raised by nonrelatives have sometimes been used as cheap labor or exploited in other ways. (Of course, some biological parents abuse their children, too.)

Styles of parenting also vary among social groups. In Western middle- and upper-class traditions, women have been expected to be married and in their late teens or 20s before they have children. In some societies, on other continents, women are expected to bear children in their teens, before marriage; in fact, they may not be considered marriageable until they have proven their fertility.

In some social groups, grandparents or other friends and relatives regularly play a major role in the care of infants and children in their families. In others, mothers are expected to cope with parenthood pretty much on their own. Though we may take the two-generation, nuclear family—two parents and their children—for granted, many other civilizations consider three or four generations under one roof to be the normal family pattern.

In some cultures, there is a "women's house" and a "men's house." In others, a whole tribe or clan lives together. Some women in North America choose to share a household and one or more children with a lover (male or female) or friends. Their other friends and relatives may consider this choice sensible, weird, or even immoral. Your decision about a problem pregnancy takes place in the context of culture and history.

In Closing

Each of us is the product of her own society and takes our society's traditions for granted. A woman who is pregnant needs to reflect on how her pregnancy and her decisions about motherhood will fit into and be received by her social subgroup, and the importance of that social acceptance in her personal values, plans, and lifestyle. Some of us are natural rebels, and some of us are miserable when we feel "different."

When you make a decision about continuing a pregnancy, the attitudes of your particular culture will have a strong influence. However, it is often helpful to reflect that those attitudes are not universal and absolute, but simply a sample of a whole wide human spectrum.

CHAPTER 3

Facts and Figures About Abortion, Birth, and Adoption

Before the 1973 *Roe v. Wade* decision by the U.S. Supreme Court legalized abortion throughout the United States, there were more than 1 million illegal abortions performed each year in our country.[1,2] Twenty percent of the deaths related to childbearing resulted from these unsafe abortions, and many other women suffered serious complications; some permanently lost their ability to have children.[3]

Now that abortion can be performed legally in medical facilities, it is among the safest surgeries performed in the United States,[4] medically safer even than childbirth itself. Data from the National Center for Health Statistics and the Centers for Disease Control and Prevention indicate that, although about 9 of every 100,000 women die during childbirth, fewer than 1 of every 100,000 die during legal abortion.[5,6]

Abortion Statistics

◆ How Common is Abortion?

About 30% of pregnancies in the United States end in abortions.[7]
Approximately 1.6 million abortions are performed each year.[8,9]
Of these abortions, 90% are performed in the first 3 months of pregnancy.[7]
These figures have held steady for the last 15 years, and if present trends continue, almost half of American women will have had an abortion by the time they reach the age of 45.[10,11]

◆ Who Has Abortions?[12]

Approximately 54% of women who have abortions are less than 25 years old.
Women in their teenage years end 38%, and women over 40 end 34%, of their pregnancies by abortion.
Of the women who have abortions, 82% are not married at the time of the procedure.
About 61% of women undergoing abortion are white.
Of women obtaining abortions, 43% have one or two children, and 45% have not had a child.
Of women who have abortions, 55% are having one for the first time.
Women who are poor are more likely to have abortions, but well-off women have abortions as well.
Although abortion is forbidden by some religious faiths (see Chapter 6), it is practiced by women of every faith.

Adoption

Statistics

Some women faced with a problem pregnancy consider adoption as one possible alternative to abortion. In the 1950s, adoption was a very popular option in the United States, especially among adolescents. During that time, as many as 80% of pregnant teenagers chose adoption.[13] Today this number has fallen to less than 5% due to the fact that most pregnant teenagers now either choose abortion or carry the child to term and raise it themselves.[13] Some older women, including those who already have one or more other children, also choose adoption, but no exact percentage is known.

Statistics about adoption are hard to come by because there is no good source of national data on this subject. Statistics must be compiled state by state from various sources such as court records, vital records, social service agency records, and estimates.[14] By this method, it is estimated that about 120,000 adoptions take place in the United States each year.[14] About half of the children who are adopted are adopted by relatives,[14] and private agencies handle most nonrelative adoptions, including up to 75% of infant adoptions.[13]

Adoption Attitudes and Opportunities

If you are considering adoption, you will want to know whether there will be a good family to take your baby. You might be considering members of your own family or people you know. This arrangement is more acceptable in some families and less acceptable in others.

Family members cannot adopt your baby against your will. It is your decision. You might feel more secure because the baby's adoptive parents will be blood relatives, because you know them, or because you will know where the baby is and how he or she is getting along. On the other hand, you and the people who adopt the baby might feel awkward: explaining the relationships and circumstances to your child as he or she grows older, or approving or disapproving of each other's lifestyles and parenting styles. You cannot and should not expect that an adoption like this can be kept a secret from your child. If family and friends refuse to talk about the adoption openly, your child will imagine that there is some shameful family secret.

If you prefer that people you don't know adopt your baby, you will use an intermediary such as a lawyer or an adoption agency. An adoption agency will check out prospective parents to see whether they have enough income, space, and stability to care for a child. They will tell you whether their records will be sealed, so that the adoptive parents and your child will not know who you are, and vice versa; whether the child will have access to the records when he or she reaches legal age; or whether the whole process can be open, with everybody knowing everybody.

Outcomes for the Mother

Much of the information about adoption comes from times when most of the women who allowed their biological children to be adopted were either unmarried or desperately poor. Abortions were unacceptable, unavailable, dangerous, and expensive. Having a baby outside marriage was considered shameful. The baby was labeled "illegitimate" on the birth certificate. The only way to escape this stigma was to be raised by another family. All of these pressures combined to make many unmarried pregnant women feel that adoption was their only alternative.

The same was true of women who were too poor to provide the bare necessities of life for a child. At the same time, society expected biological mothers to be attached to their children; giving up a child meant, both to the mother and to others in society, that she did not love the child as she should. These attitudes have not completely disappeared from our society. They still have an influence on women who have their children adopted.

Because adoptions traditionally took place under circumstances in which the pregnancy and birth were taboo subjects, most of the women involved did not reveal this personal history and could not be followed up by scientists studying the outcome of adoption. The only women who have made their feelings public are some of those who regret their decisions to give up their children. There is no way to know to what degree these women are representative of others whose children have been adopted.

Outcomes for the Child

Adoption was a closely guarded family secret until a generation ago, when experts began to recommend that adoptive parents talk openly with their children about how they came into the family. Experts in child development believed that adopted children had special difficulties in establishing a sense of identity and were more vulnerable to emotional disturbances than were children brought up by their biological parents.

More recent studies show that the impact of adoption depends a great deal on the circumstances. What is a child told about the reasons for the adoption? How do the adoptive parents feel about their inability to have biological children, or their decision to add a child to their family through adoption rather than birth? No one's life is without conflicts, and adopted children have the advantage of knowing that they are very much wanted by their adoptive parents.

Trends in Adoption

Traditionally, adoption agencies kept the biological and adoptive parents apart from one another. The biological mother was expected to cut all ties to her child and to get on with her life. This protected her from exposure of a potentially humiliating history and protected the adoptive family from intrusion. In recent years, new attitudes and trends have emerged. There are organizations both for and against giving adopted children the opportunity to meet their biological parents. In open adoption, the biological and adoptive parents meet before the birth, get to know each other, and share each other's lives and, to some degree, the child. Sometimes the prospective adoptive parents offer the pregnant woman financial support and attend the birth.

These new kinds of relationships, like the traditional ones, have both advantages and disadvantages. On one hand, the adoptive parents are often more financially and socially secure than the biological parent(s). Knowing this, the biological mother can be reassured that her child has been placed into a loving family who is well able to meet the needs of the child. On the other hand, she may feel jealous because the new family has advantages she can't enjoy. And the biological and adoptive parents may have little in common with each other except for the child, making their interactions difficult or awkward.

There are no scientific studies to inform us which styles of adoption are better for mothers or their children. If you are considering adoption, you will need to find out what styles are available in your geographic area, and to reflect carefully about which would work out better for you—not only now, but also in the long run, when your life circumstances change.

The Adoption Process

Although there is considerable publicity about the shortage of children for childless couples to adopt, that situation applies only to healthy white babies. Adoption agencies set standards for adoptive parents. These standards may include age, income, religion, lifestyle, and family stability. People who do not meet these criteria are sometimes allowed to adopt children who would otherwise not find homes: older, physically or mentally ill, disabled, or multiracial children. A court of law must formalize each adoption. Practices and standards vary widely. For example, some homosexual adults have been allowed to adopt children.[19] Others have lost custody of their biological children because they were homosexual.

Adoption across racial lines is also controversial. The advantages of a stable home must be weighed against problems that could arise because parents and child are of different races. Some leaders of minority groups feel that the adoption of minority children of needy parents by more affluent, white families is exploitation. They believe that children should be raised in their own racial culture, with a clear racial history and identity, and prepared for the realities of life as a member of their own race. On the other hand, limiting the placement of children to families of the same race can be interpreted as racist; many people have mixed racial heritage, and a child is a child, whatever the color.

You can get information about adoption from a child welfare or adoption agency in your community. Some adoptions are also arranged privately. A local member of the clergy, a lawyer, or a physician may know of prospective adoptive parents. Prospective adoptive parents also advertise in major newspapers, with private attorneys to make the legal arrangements. You will want to consider which issues are most important to you: the stability and services of an adoption agency, or the opportunity for personal contact and choice of a private adoption.

Local laws and practices determine the amount of contact the mother has with her child before the baby is given to the adoptive parents, whether the infant is cared for by a foster family or agency for some period before going home with the adoptive parents, and at what point the adoption becomes legal and permanent. Lawmakers and judges must weigh the right of the birth mother to consider and reconsider her decision with the rights of the adoptive parents and the infant to establish a secure family without worrying that the birth mother may change her mind and take the baby back.

Becoming a Parent

What Can You Expect?

All of us have been children, and all of us have observed others as children and as parents. Those experiences may make you determined to do certain things and avoid others when you are a parent. On the other hand, everything may feel different when it is you who is pregnant. You may not be sure what staying pregnant and becoming a parent would be like for you.

Most pregnant women in the United States continue their pregnancies and keep and care for their babies. The experiences, successes, and failures of parenting are incredibly varied. People often are surprised or dismayed by a pregnancy but grow to accept and welcome it. Parenting a child is perhaps life's greatest challenge and, under many circumstances, life's greatest joy. Although there are people who regret having had a child, they generally feel uncomfortable talking about their regrets, so we don't have scientific information about how many there are.

There is scientific information about the effect of motherhood on women's educations, the kinds of jobs they get, and their satisfaction with their lives. In general, all of these effects are negative. But many of the joys and pains of parenting cannot be reduced to numbers.[15] How can we weigh the joy of a toddler's hug or a teenager's graduation against an advanced degree or a high-level career position never attained?

Another consideration is the uncertainty of any pregnancy's outcome. If you have a child, he or she could have a physical or mental disability or could grow up to be a genius or a great athlete. Even with prenatal testing, there is no way to rule out all possibility of birth defects.

Pregnant Teenagers

Some people think the solution for a teenager's problem pregnancy is marriage. But marriage does not guarantee a supportive environment for motherhood, especially for a young teenager. In fact, marriage of a pregnant teenager is associated with a greater probability of her leaving school and becoming, or remaining, poor in adulthood.[16,17]

With the help of supportive families, some adolescent mothers can care adequately for themselves and a child. The birth of a second child, though, makes it much more likely that a teenage mother will never finish school, will be poor all of her life, and will not be able to provide an adequate environment for her children.[18] One recent review of research on teenage pregnancy indicates that one-quarter of all young women in the United States today have been pregnant by the time they reached age 18. Of those women ages 15–19 who gave birth in 1988, 83% were poor or had low incomes. Adolescent mothers were more likely to be receiving public assistance than were women who delayed childbearing until their early 20s. In addition, only 70% of teenage mothers finish high school by age 39, whereas 90% of older mothers finish by that time.[18]

Parenthood When Abortion Is Denied

There are studies from Czechoslovakia and Denmark of women who wanted abortions but couldn't get them. Because these countries had national health care systems with detailed record-keeping, the requests, denials, and outcomes of these cases have been documented. Abortion was legal but required official authorization in these countries. Children who were born after their mothers had been denied abortion were compared with other, control children, born at the same time, whose mothers had not applied for abortions. The children of mothers denied abortions did more poorly in school and were more likely to get into trouble with the law than was true for the control children.[19,20]

Some of these studies have now extended for as long as 30 years. Over those years, many other influences have been added to the effect of the mothers' preferences. At this point, the differences between the two groups have almost disappeared.[19]

Studies such as these do not indicate that some people should never have been born. They do indicate that children born despite their mothers' requests for abortion may need special support from society during their childhood and young adulthood.

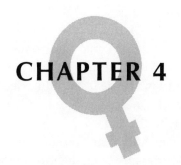

CHAPTER 4

State and National Abortion Laws and Regulations

Because laws and regulations affecting abortion are constantly changing on national and state levels, this book does not list the specific laws and regulations for every geographic area. To obtain that information, you can call the national or local office of the organizations listed at the end of this chapter. In this chapter, I discuss the development of abortion law in general, several major U.S. Supreme Court decisions affecting abortion nationwide, and some of the arguments for and against specific abortion regulations as they may affect you.

Abortion Law in U.S. History

Abortion was outlawed in the United States only about 100 years ago. Before that time, the laws did not concern themselves with abortion one way or the other. Most reproductive health care for women was provided by other women in the community—midwives who were not medically trained but who learned their trade from those who came before. As the profession of medicine became increasingly structured and regulated, obstetrics and gynecology became a medical specialty, and childbirth became a medical event.

Official medical organizations stated that childbirth was a woman's duty. Under increasing pressure from doctors, both contraception and abortion were limited by state laws. The taboo surrounding both forced women to go "underground" to obtain them, if they could, and thus set up a vicious circle. The trauma that women experienced in the process of obtaining illegal abortions contributed to the sense that abortion was a shameful and dangerous procedure.

As the 20th century progressed, the laws banning contraceptives were challenged in the courts by health care workers and social activists, who were horrified by the suffering and danger of repeated childbearing and illegal abortions, specifically, the losses to families when sisters and mothers suffered hemorrhages, infections, and death. One by one, states overturned the laws barring contraceptives. Some held out until the middle of the 20th century. Soon after, some states began to reconsider their positions on abortion.

During the 1960s, New York and a few other states legalized abortion. Women began flocking from all over the country to New York to terminate pregnancies legally and safely.

Roe v. Wade

In 1972, a Texas woman ("Roe" was not her real name but rather was the name used in the court case to protect her identity) became pregnant under difficult circumstances and wanted an abortion. She challenged the Texas law forbidding abortions in court on the grounds that the prohibition of abortion deprived her of the right to privacy. The Supreme Court had previously decided that this right was guaranteed by the liberty clause of the Bill of Rights of the U.S. Constitution. Henry Wade, the other party in the case, was the Dallas County prosecutor opposing Roe's claim. The case progressed to the U.S. Supreme Court, where it was decided, as *Roe v. Wade,* in 1973. The Supreme Court struck down state abortion bans, legalizing abortion throughout the United States on the grounds of women's right to privacy.

The Hyde Amendment

The *Roe v. Wade* decision has precipitated an ongoing battle by groups opposing abortion. The battle continues today, taking many forms and being fought on many legal battlefields. Representative Henry Hyde of Illinois introduced and passed an amendment in the U.S. Congress in 1976 that forbids the use of federal funds to pay for abortions. Thus, many women who are poor and who rely on national programs for their health care cannot obtain abortions, despite the fact that they are legal. This limitation has been challenged in courts around the country but has not been eliminated.

Challenges to *Roe v. Wade*

As successive Supreme Court justices retire and are replaced, changing the composition of the Court, cases are repeatedly brought before the Court to challenge the standing *Roe v. Wade* decision. Three of the most important cases have been *Webster v. Reproductive Health Services* in 1989, *Casey v. Planned Parenthood* in 1992, and *Akron v. Akron Center for Reproductive Health* in 1983. Although Supreme Court decisions may apply directly only in a particular situation or to a particular state or municipality, their implications are national. The opinion of the Supreme Court on one state's law influences all the other states and municipalities that are contemplating laws and regulations of their own. Often new laws are written in the same terms, or with the same provisions, that the Court has approved in a previous case.

The *Webster* case concerned a Missouri state law (the parties in the case are a state official and a facility where abortions were performed) that banned the performance of abortions in public medical facilities and by public employees, except when the woman's medical condition made her pregnancy an immediate risk to her life. (Because of improvements in obstetric care, such situations are increasingly rare.)

The Missouri law also prohibits the use of public funds "to advise or counsel a woman to have an abortion." There is no specific definition of this phrase.

Health care workers helping women think through reproductive decisions run the risk of violating this law. Many kinds of health care facilities receive some form of public support. Some health care providers may not be sure whether "public funds" are being used in their work with particular patients. Concerns about violating the law thus intrude into care, which should be focused on patients.

The law also requires physicians to perform complicated laboratory tests, regardless of whether they are needed for the medical care of the woman, if she might be 20 or more weeks pregnant. The tests are meant to determine whether the fetus has any chance for life outside the woman's body. The Supreme Court allows the physician to determine whether the tests are necessary. However, doctors may feel that they had better order these expensive tests in every case, because of fears of legal liability.

Lastly, the Court allowed the following wording in the Missouri law: "the life of each human being begins at conception," and "unborn children have protected interests in life, health and well-being." These statements are extremely controversial—philosophically, biologically, and legally. Some embryos and fetuses grow into people, and others do not, regardless of whether an abortion takes place. An embryo or a fetus has the potential to become a person, but it is not capable of life on its own. Some people believe it is already a person, and some don't. American legal tradition has not recognized anyone as a person until that person is born.

The *Casey* decision concerned several other barriers to abortion. The law enacted in Pennsylvania required that married women obtain their husbands' consent for abortions and that women under the age of legal majority obtain consent from their parents. It required a waiting period of 24 hours or more between the time a woman asked a doctor for an abortion and the time she was allowed to have the procedure. It also required that certain specific statements be provided to the woman both orally and in writing. This communication to a pregnant woman had to be made regardless of whether it was scientifically accurate, whether the woman wanted to hear it, whether she could understand it, or how it would affect her psychologically. The statements include descriptions of embryos at various stages of development and claims about the availability of obstetric care and financial child support in Pennsylvania.

Of course, women should have whatever information they want and need. Women should be able to discuss their decisions with people they love and trust. But these requirements were not intended to inform or protect women, but to make it more difficult for them to have abortions. If you are given information like this—information you haven't asked for—it's probably because you live in a state with a law like this.

The *Casey* decision did support the basic theory of *Roe v. Wade*—the privacy right of women to abortion. This aspect of the decision made all the headlines. The Supreme Court also overturned the requirement for a husband's consent. But the Court upheld the requirements for the specific statements to the woman seeking an abortion, for parents' consent for young women's abortions, and for a waiting period. The Supreme Court declared that states could enact "reasonable" restrictions on abortion. Aside from allowing the restrictions specified in the Pennsylvania law, the Court did not define "reasonable." That definition is highly controversial.

Finally, the *Akron* case was an earlier case in which the Court also upheld a requirement of parental consent for minors wishing to obtain abortions. However, the court also decided that minors who were sufficiently mature to make the decision on their own, and who had good reasons for not seeking parental consent, should be able to obtain approval for an abortion from a judge in a process known as "judicial bypass." In addition, the *Akron* decision stated that states with parental consent laws were to establish procedures to guarantee that the process of obtaining a judicial bypass would be quick and confidential.

The Impact of Legal Restrictions

This section presents a discussion of the effects of these state laws and Supreme Court decisions on actual pregnant women. Are headlines accurate when they claim that the right to abortion has been protected?

Does a right mean anything if you or other women can't exercise it?

Laws restricting abortion have definitely decreased the numbers of legal abortions performed in the United States. The number of pregnancies has not decreased, so the number of births has increased. Presumably, some of the additional women who give birth would have had abortions if it were not for the restrictions. Some women are mothers, and some babies have been born, because of these restrictions. Is that good or bad? It depends on the circumstances and your point of view.

Another result of restrictive laws is that illegal abortions seem to have returned to the geographic areas where the restrictions apply. We can't expect women who had illegal abortions to report them to the authorities for statistical records, but there are certain kinds of injuries and infections that are almost always the result of illegal abortions. Women with those injuries and infections do have to come to hospitals for care, where those complications can be observed. They are a good indication that illegal abortions are taking place.

There is no scientific evidence that restrictions on legal abortions have had the other protective effects on women and families that they are supposed to have had. There is no evidence that they have increased family communication or closeness, have made abortion decisions more informed or thoughtful, or have made abortion more safe.

Discrimination Against Public Institutions and Their Patients

Many women receive their health care from public institutions, whether for reasons of geographic availability or financial necessity. Limitations on abortion in publicly funded hospitals and clinics limit their care. These restrictions also prevent medical and nursing trainees in public institutions from learning to counsel women who may be considering abortions and from learning to perform abortions.

Interference in the Doctor-Patient Relationship

Government-mandated speeches interfere with the freedom of a doctor and a patient to choose a style of communication that is comfortable and comprehensible for both of them, as is legally required for in-formed consent. In no other situation in medicine is a doctor legally or professionally required to speak to a patient in specific words. There is no evidence that a lack of information about prenatal development, prenatal care, and laws requiring fathers to provide child support inter-fered with women's ability to make decisions about their pregnancies.

Interference by Husbands and Parents: Risks of Abuse

Laws that give people other than the pregnant woman control over her pregnancy intrude on her rights in a way that is not allowed under any other circumstances. The law does not permit any invasion, no matter how minor, of one person's body for the benefit, no matter how critical, of another person. For example, no one can be forced to donate blood for another person, even when the donation is no risk to the donor and the blood is necessary to save the life of the other person. The potential donor cannot be forced to consult with anyone in particular or to re-ceive particular information. No one else has any say in the decision.

Obviously a husband has a stake in his wife's pregnancy. But should he have a legal right to decide whether she can have an abortion? When a wife and husband have a healthy relationship, they will choose to discuss important decisions. Most pregnant married women care a great deal about their husbands' feelings and preferences. But a woman's husband may be abusive, threatening, or absent. That may well be the reason she is considering an abortion.

The issues for women under legal age are related, but somewhat dif-ferent. What is similar is the interest of another person, in this case the parent, in the outcome of the pregnancy. The difference is the tradi-tional right of parents to make medical decisions for their minor chil-dren. The courts have also recognized the rights of adolescents, especially those who have left—or have been left by—their families to lead independent lives, to make or participate in decisions about their own medical care. Adolescents who assume responsibility for them-selves are legally considered "emancipated."

Adolescents who become pregnant have the legal right to make de-cisions about obstetric care and procedures, such as the performance of cesarean deliveries. When they become mothers, they are legally entitled to make decisions about their children's medical care, even when their own parents still have authority over their medical care. Court decisions in some states, such as California, have held that abortion must be treated like other medical decisions related to pregnancy. If an adolescent mother can decide to let her child have open-heart surgery, and a pregnant adolescent can decide to have a cesarean birth, then a pregnant adolescent can also decide to have an abortion.

Most pregnant adolescents discuss their pregnancy decisions with their parents.[1] The younger the woman, the more likely she is to involve her parents.[2] Physicians providing care for adolescents help them involve their parents in major decisions whenever it is in the adolescents' best interest. Loving, competent parents know their daughters' personalities, circumstances, values, and plans for the future. They help their daughters think through their options, and they support their decisions.

However, there are important reasons why parental involvement, whether for consultation or consent, should not be legally required. Like some married couples, some families are dysfunctional. Some young women are victims of incest; sexual, physical, or emotional abuse; or severe parental neglect. In fact, young women in these circumstances are more likely to become pregnant than young women in healthier families. Some young women have good reason to believe that their pregnancies would precipitate a family breakdown. They and/or others would be beaten or thrown out of the family household. Their hopes for a normal education and a decent future would be destroyed. Their parents might refuse consent, forcing them to go through with the pregnancy and childbirth and to become mothers against their will.

Laws requiring parents' notification or consent assume that all parents are mature and responsible and have the best interests of their daughters at heart. No parental consent is required in order for the pregnant young woman to continue her pregnancy and take on all the rights and responsibilities of motherhood. It makes sense that a young woman who has the legal right to take on the responsibilities of motherhood should also have the legal right to decide not to assume those responsibilities.

Judicial Bypass

The Supreme Court has ruled that laws requiring parental notification or consent for abortion must make an exception for young women who are victims of child abuse or incest. This exception is called *judicial bypass*. This process was first specified in the case of *Hodgson v. Minnesota* in 1990. A judicial bypass allows a young woman to come to court and face a judge, describe her situation, and argue that she is "emancipated"—mature enough to make a decision for herself—or that her parents are neglectful, absent, or abusive and not able to play a constructive role in her decision making.

Judicial bypass of parental consent is neither realistic nor fair. First of all, how is a pregnant adolescent to know that there is such a thing as a judicial bypass? There is no way to provide this information to all the young women who need it.

Once a young woman does learn about judicial bypass, what does she have to do to get one? She must find out which court is in charge of this particular process among the bewildering array of courts and judges: federal, state, county, and city. She must get to the court. Because she feels that it is not advisable or safe to advise her parents of her pregnancy, she must find an acceptable explanation for her absence for a time long enough to get back and forth to court, wait, and have a court hearing. Most courts are in session during normal school and working hours, and not at other times. She must do all of this while in the midst of a life crisis and under time pressure to make and implement a major decision.

Her problems don't end when she gets to court. Although judicial bypass statutes require that the judicial proceeding be confidential, she will have to tell courthouse personnel her business so that she can ask for directions to the right courtroom. She also may be seen and heard by members of the community who have other business in the building. They may wonder, or surmise, what an adolescent is doing there. They may well know her, her family, her teachers, and others she might wish not to know about her situation. People or groups opposed to abortion may attempt to approach, pressure, or harass her, further increasing her stress.

In many cases, local court judges hold hearings in a given court only on specific days. She may arrive only to learn that the designated judge is not available. She may have to make her excuses, miss school or job time, and find transportation again, while living with a pregnancy she does not want as it progresses from day to day and week to week. One of the most common causes of abortion after the first 3 months of pregnancy is the inability to obtain an abortion during the first 3 months.[3]

Throughout this process, the pregnant adolescent faces an awesome prospect: standing in a court of law in front of a judge. A court is a frightening place for most people, even when they are not young, not in the midst of a difficult life circumstance, and not forced to plead for a procedure that is critical for their immediate and long-term future. Many people who have been abused or neglected are ashamed and intimidated. It often takes them years to reveal their histories of abuse to a trusted friend or therapist. The young woman in this situation must make a convincing case and come across as mature enough to make an independent decision.

Judicial bypass procedures have been practiced for several years, and information is now available about their use and the outcomes. Judges' decisions in these cases vary widely among states. In some states, nearly every young woman who seeks a judicial bypass is granted one, and in others, nearly every young woman is denied one. That is not fair.

The Real Burdens of Waiting Periods

State laws requiring waiting periods before an abortion can be performed have been approved by the Supreme Court. These requirements are supposed to ensure that women have time to think it over before having abortions. However, the scientific evidence indicates that women do think about their decisions very carefully before arranging to have abortions.

The real impact of waiting periods comes from the uneven geographic distribution of abortion providers. Eighty percent of the counties in the United States currently have no abortion provider at all. Two large states in the United States currently have one or no provider.[4] In some regions of the country, particularly in the Midwest, the number of abortion providers has actually decreased during the past two decades.[5] A waiting period requirement means that a woman has to come to a clinic, request an abortion, and then return for a second visit after the required waiting period. She must either travel twice or stay overnight or longer. Travel, overnight stays, and meals away from home cost money and disrupt jobs, school, and family responsibilities. Some abortion clinics are open only one or more days of the week because the personnel travel over a geographic area or work elsewhere on the other days. A 1-day legislated wait may mean a week's wait in practical terms.

For a wealthy woman, these requirements can be minor or major inconveniences. For a poor woman, they can mean having to choose between buying immediate family essentials, such as food for the family, and the abortion. They can force her to leave her children in a makeshift care situation. For any woman, the waiting period, with its double travel or overnight stay(s), requires that she find an acceptable explanation for her absences from her job, school, and family. It makes it more difficult to keep this personal and intimate decision confidential. For a woman who is the victim of domestic violence, that may mean the inability to have the abortion that she has decided is necessary, as well as possible psychological abuse, battering, or death.

Limitations on Medical Care

In addition to laws in each individual state, there is existing and pending national legislation on abortion. The Hyde Amendment, named after its author, U.S. Representative Henry Hyde of Illinois, was passed by Congress in 1976 as a compromise between pro- and anti-choice forces and prohibits the use of federal funds for abortions. Mr. Hyde's argument in favor of his amendment was that he and many other American taxpayers were morally opposed to abortions and should not have to pay for them. But we don't use that reasoning about other taxes; we have to pay our taxes whether or not we agree with the way they're spent. It is not a matter of economy, either, because federal funds are used to pay for the obstetric care of needy women who cannot obtain abortions, as well as for the medical care of the children who are born. Each of these costs very much more than an abortion.[6]

Many of the women whose circumstances make them vulnerable to unintended pregnancy face significant financial barriers to obtaining abortions. A "right" is just a word if people cannot exercise it in the real world. The Hyde Amendment does not affect individual states, which may choose whether or not to use state funds to pay for the abortions of medically indigent women. Some states, such as California, provide state funds for the reproductive health care of medically indigent people, leaving it to individual women and their health care providers to decide what type of care—abortion or childbirth—is best in each case.

Another barrier to abortion is so-called "conscience clauses" in some health care legislation. Health care systems have been undergoing a major upheaval in the United States. Many health care providers and consumers have joined large, structured, managed health care organizations. The state and federal governments, concerned about the costs of health care for the poor and the elderly, and about the gaps in health care insurance for the rest of the population, have also enacted regulations about medical care. A "conscience clause" in a law or regulation means that no state-funded institution or health care provider is required to offer care that violates its "conscience." Many health care systems are run by religious groups, and some of these groups oppose abortion. When the state mandates the enrollment of all medically indigent individuals into managed health care systems, a woman may not be able to choose a health care provider who will mention, discuss, refer her for, or perform an abortion.

Harassment and Violence

Recently, there have been new approaches to the legal protection of freedom of choice. In some parts of the country, abortion is legal and available in abortion clinics. However, anti-abortion groups demonstrate at these clinics. The demonstrators, convinced that their aims justify nearly any means, confront, accuse, and plead with women who are trying to obtain medical care. The protestors physically block vehicles and pedestrians entering clinic grounds, shove frightening pamphlets and photographs through open car windows and into people's hands, and shout in their ears. Many abortion clinics have been vandalized or destroyed and staff members intentionally injured and even killed. Needless to say, these incidents terrorize other staff, patients, and friends and relatives who accompany women they care about.

In some places, professionals involved in abortion care have been targeted for demonstrations and harassment in the other places where they work and their neighborhoods. Their children have been taunted at school that their parents "murder" babies. The abortion laws in some states specify that the names, addresses, and telephone numbers of doctors who perform abortions and women who have abortions must be supplied to the state. There is no such requirement for any other medical procedure. These requirements allow anti-abortion groups to trace, contact, and harass the women and doctors who receive and perform abortions. Even where there are laws forbidding these activities, those laws are enforced in some places and ignored in others.

Currently, there are efforts to outlaw clinic vandalism, harassment, and obstruction. There are two relevant Supreme Court decisions. In *Bray v. Alexandria Women's Health Clinic,* a 1993 decision, the Court ruled that clinic anti-abortion protests do not violate the Civil Rights Act because the women attending the clinics did not legally constitute a "group," or class of people who were discriminated against and therefore required federal civil rights protection. However, in *National Organization for Women v. Scheidler,* in 1994, the Supreme Court decided that anti-abortion groups whose protests interfered with or prevented the operation of legitimate businesses—that is, abortion clinics—could be prosecuted under the Racketeer-Influenced and Corrupt Organizations (RICO) Law.

Protecting Reproductive Choice

Some laws guarantee freedom of choice rather than limit it. Bills guaranteeing freedom of choice have been introduced in the federal, and some state, legislatures. The state of Maryland, for example, has enacted such a bill into law. The purpose of freedom-of-choice laws is to emphasize the citizens' support for choice and to remove legal access to abortion from the unpredictable control of court decisions. At the same time, medical educators have launched efforts to reduce the shortage of abortion providers through the training of family practitioners and obstetrician-gynecologists to perform abortions.

For Further Information

The information provided here about abortion laws in various states is the latest available when the book went to press. Up-to-the-minute data are available from organizations such as the Alan Guttmacher Institute, the American Civil Liberties Union's Reproductive Freedom Project, the Planned Parenthood Federation of America, and the Center for Reproductive Law and Policy. The addresses and telephone numbers of these organizations are listed in the Resource Directory at the end of this book.

Several of these organizations publish newsletters or other resources to which you can subscribe. You may wish to know what the laws are because they directly affect you or someone you love, or because you want to participate in the legislative or judicial process. It is important to know not only which laws are in effect at a given moment, but also whether there are bills under consideration in the national or state legislature, or laws that are "on the books" but are not being enforced because they are undergoing court review. These organizations may also be able to help you to find alternatives, to get funding, or to support or challenge laws in the legislatures and courts.

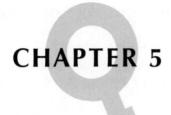

CHAPTER 5

Abortion Procedures

This chapter outlines the current range of abortion practices in order to help you think about your personal preferences and ask informed questions in the health care setting. As a consumer, you must always weigh your preferences against the range of services actually available to you; the experience, skill, and attitudes of the medical staff who will perform the abortion; and the possibility that some aspect of your health will require one particular form of abortion procedure rather than another. You are always somewhat handicapped by the fact that medical professionals may know—or insist they know—more about the decision than you can understand, or may be unable to explain their advice or practice to your satisfaction. Again, you have to weigh your right to information and choice against time constraints and the risks of arguing with the staff who are actually available to perform your abortion.

Your Right to Information

The single most important fact about abortion procedures is that you are entitled to information about any procedure you are considering.

The Ideal Situation

Under the best of circumstances, you would be able to go to the clinic or other medical facility ahead of time in order to meet with the staff there, see the facility, get information about the process, and ask whatever questions you may have. Your questions would be clear in your mind, and you would be able to express them clearly. The clinic personnel would be respectful, relaxed, and informative. If anyone did seem insensitive, you would command respect by sticking to your questions politely but firmly. You would also be able to bring along one or two other people who are supportive: your spouse, lover, friend, or relative. They would be able to ask questions about the abortion and about how they can best help you before, during, and after the procedure.

Other Situations

Real life, however, seldom lives up to ideals. You may live far away from the clinic, or it may be open on only a limited schedule. Your time may be limited by family or job demands. You may have to do some of your fact-finding over the telephone or at the same visit as the abortion itself. You may have to, or want to, do it alone.

Your own feelings may also restrict your access to information. Many of us are reluctant to ask, even politely, for the time of medical professionals. Doctors and nurses always look busy.

Some of us feel overwhelmed in a medical setting and have difficulty putting our thoughts and feelings into words. Many of us have unpleasant memories of past medical experiences. The prospect of having another medical procedure adds to our anxiety. That other person who may have agreed to come along, but who is not personally facing a medical procedure, can be enormously helpful in asking the questions you want answered—but only if that person knows what you want to know and is not too preoccupied with his or her own feelings.

Counseling

Counseling is offered by most facilities where abortions are performed. Abortion counseling is not the same as giving information to a patient so that she can give informed consent. Informed consent means that a person has been given, and has understood, *information* about the nature of a proposed procedure or treatment, its risks and benefits, and the alternatives and their risks and benefits and that she has *consented* to have the procedure. Counseling goes beyond that information to include a discussion of the woman's personal preferences, situation, and feelings. The counselor and the woman should review the reasons the woman wants the abortion, what she knows about it, what her support system is, and how she expects her decision to affect her.

Although the decision of whether to have an abortion still belongs to the woman herself, the counselor may point out areas the woman does not seem to have considered. She (nearly all counselors are women[1]) has been trained to notice when a woman seems much more upset than other women planning an abortion. She will help the woman decide whether she needs to calm down, think a bit more, or consult with other people before proceeding with the abortion. The counselor may offer to meet with the woman and whomever else is closely involved in order to help them discuss the decision together.

There is some disagreement about requiring a woman to have counseling before she can have an abortion. Requiring—rather than simply offering—counseling implies that women are not able to make the decision on their own, involving those they choose to advise and support them. Without any evidence, it picks out abortion as a special problem, as compared with other medical procedures and other life decisions. No counseling is required, for instance, when a woman decides to continue a pregnancy and deliver a baby. No counseling is required before most major surgery. Those in favor of required counseling see it as a helpful intervention, to ensure that a woman considers every factor she should before acting on her decision and to give her support.

There are so-called "counseling centers" that are really set up to attract pregnant women so as to pressure them not to have abortions. Their names may be misleading. Counseling should not push you strongly in any particular direction. If a center is run by a religious or other group opposed to abortion, the staff should tell you so. If you find yourself being pressured, just leave. You may want to report the center to the state department of public health.

Genuine abortion counselors may be social workers, psychologists, family counselors, or volunteers who have offered to learn about abortion in order to help other women. Abortion counselors vary in style and approach, but every counselor should help the woman to think through her situation, including her religious beliefs; her financial resources; her living arrangements; her family, academic, and career goals; and her relationships with lovers, parents, other relatives, and friends. The pregnant woman and the counselor will also discuss the options and how the woman might expect them to play out over the coming weeks, months, and years. Discussion with a neutral, informed, and helpful third party can help a person to see things from different perspectives or to realize possibilities she had not considered. Although few women change their plans as a result of abortion counseling, most women find it helpful.

Questions You May Have

Most women thinking about abortion want to know:

- The medical risks and complications
- Whether there will be pain
- What method of anesthesia will be used
- How long the process takes
- How long it will be before they can return to their usual activities
- What warning signs they should watch for after the abortion
- Which staff members will be present during the abortion

- Who will perform the abortion
- Whether the procedure will be kept confidential

Risk Factors Related to the Stage of Pregnancy

Abortion procedures used, as well as the risk of complications, change as pregnancy advances. The length of a pregnancy is often described in 3-month intervals, or *trimesters*. Three trimesters add up to the 9 months of pregnancy. Pregnancy is dated from the beginning of a woman's last normal menstrual period. If a woman has a 28-day cycle, she is considered to be 4 weeks pregnant when her last period was 4 weeks before.

At any stage of pregnancy, abortion is associated with fewer medical complications than full-term delivery of a child.[2] The rate of complications is fewer than 1 in 100 women who have abortions in the first trimester, and 2 in 100 who undergo abortions later in pregnancy. The risk of death from first-trimester abortion is less than 1 per 100,000 abortions. This is approximately $\frac{1}{10}$ the risk of death from childbirth.[2,3]

Abortion Procedures

Abortion procedures fall into three categories:

1. Surgical
2. Induction of labor
3. Antiprogesterones

Surgical Abortion Procedures

Four kinds of abortion procedures are considered surgical:

1. Menstrual regulation or extraction
2. Vacuum suction

3. Dilatation and evacuation
4. Hysterotomy or hysterectomy

Menstrual regulation or extraction is the suctioning out of the contents of the uterus when a woman's menstrual period is due. It does not require that pregnancy has been diagnosed. A soft, narrow, sterile plastic tube is inserted through the natural opening in the cervix, and suction is applied. The process causes some cramping discomfort but does not require anesthesia.

Vacuum or *suction* curettage is by far the most common abortion procedure, used in approximately 95% of all abortions.[4] Suction is most often used for first-trimester abortions. The entire procedure takes about 10 minutes.

The woman lies in stirrups on an operating table, as she would for a pelvic examination. A vaginal speculum is inserted to hold the walls of the vagina apart so that the cervix (the lower opening of the uterus) can be seen by the doctor or nurse practitioner. This does not cause any pain. Next, the cervix and upper vaginal region are washed with an antiseptic solution, and a local anesthetic is administered to numb the cervix. General anesthesia is normally not used during a suction curettage because it is considered unnecessary and can actually increase the risk of complications or death, as with any surgical procedure.[5]

After the cervix is numbed, it is held steady with a clamp. The cervical opening is gradually dilated, or widened, with sterile dilators until it is large enough for a flexible plastic tube, called a *cannula,* to be inserted. The tube is inserted into the uterus and then attached to a vacuum device. Suction is applied, and the tissues that make up the pregnancy are removed from the uterus. The actual suctioning portion of the procedure lasts about 2–5 minutes.[6] After the vacuuming procedure, the doctor or nurse practitioner may remove the tube and insert another instrument to explore the uterine cavity to make sure it is empty.

An alternative approach is dilation and curettage (D&C). In this procedure, a sharp instrument, called a *curette,* is used to remove the contents of the uterus after the cervix has been dilated. D&Cs are also performed for other medical purposes. Normally, however, the use of suction is preferred for abortion because it involves less time, less blood loss, and fewer complications than sharp curettage.[5]

Dilation and evacuation (D&E) is the surgical technique most often used in second-trimester abortions.[6] It is generally used for pregnancies at 13–16 weeks but can be used up to 21 weeks.[6] During a D&E, the cervix is dilated in a way similar to that during a suction curettage. The contents of the uterus are then removed with both an electrical vacuum tool and an instrument called *forceps*—a long, thin, metal, tweezer-like instrument that is used to grasp the contents of the uterus. The evacuation takes about 10–15 minutes. Most often, a general anesthetic is used during D&E, but on some occasions a local anesthetic may be used.

Finally, some second- or third-trimester abortions are performed through hysterotomy or hysterectomy. A hysterotomy involves making a surgical incision into the uterus in order to remove the tissues making up the pregnancy—somewhat like a small cesarean section. A hysterectomy involves removing all or part of the uterus, along with its contents. Such procedures are hardly ever used, because the surgical techniques involved are much more complex than those used in other surgical abortion procedures and the rate of complications is much higher.[6]

Induction of Labor

Third-trimester and late second-trimester abortions are medically performed like premature deliveries. They can be done with surgery or by inducing contractions of the uterus, like labor. One such procedure is the injection of a salt (saline), or urea, solution into the uterus. This results in both the death of the fetus and the initiation of labor. More commonly, medications called *prostaglandins* are used. These are substances that occur naturally in the body and are involved in natural, spontaneous labor. Medications to induce labor can be placed into the vagina or injected into the uterus or into a vein through an intravenous line. After the labor-stimulating treatment is given, labor generally begins within 12 hours, and the abortion itself occurs within 12 hours after that.

These kinds of abortions are most often performed in general hospitals. The methods of pain relief that are available during these procedures are similar to those used for full-term labor. Most often, a local anesthetic is used for the injection site itself, and painkillers are given during the labor and delivery stages. Although abortions involving the induction of labor are medically safe—and safer than full-term delivery—they require a longer period of care and are associated with more complications than abortions performed in the first trimester.[3] The medications used to initiate labor may cause nausea, vomiting, diarrhea, and/or fever in some women. Sometimes the expulsion of the fetus is not followed immediately by the expulsion of the placenta, or "afterbirth." In this case, instruments are used to empty the uterus 1–2 hours after the abortion itself. Many women also experience severe uterine cramps and gastrointestinal discomfort after prostaglandin injections.

Antiprogesterones

Antiprogesterones are medications taken orally to induce abortion. The most common of these medications is the drug RU-486, which is widely used throughout Europe. This drug has been the source of much controversy in the United States and is not generally available. Antiprogesterones have success rates of 60%–85% when used alone.[7] Their effectiveness can be increased through the use of multiple doses or by combining antiprogesterones with prostaglandins. One study has demonstrated a 94% success rate for antiprogesterones when combined with prostaglandins in terminating early pregnancy.[7]

The most common side effect of antiprogesterones is heavy bleeding (as heavy as, or heavier than, that occurring during a normal menstrual period) lasting an average of $1\frac{1}{2}$ weeks.[7] Fatigue, nausea, headaches, and abdominal cramps are also common. Finally, if the abortion attempt is incomplete or unsuccessful—meaning that all of the tissues making up the pregnancy were not completely removed—vacuum curettage is required to remove the remaining pregnancy tissues from the uterus (see the section "Complications" later in this chapter).

Early Versus Late Abortions

Most abortions are performed early in pregnancy in a clinic or doctor's office. As already mentioned, suction curettage is the most common procedure used for these early abortions. Early abortions tend to be less expensive, to involve a shorter period of recovery, and to have fewer potential complications than later abortions—those performed in the second or third trimester.

However, there are many reasons why some women seek late abortions. Some may not have realized that they were pregnant until the pregnancy had already progressed beyond the first trimester. Others may have had difficulty finding an abortion provider or obtaining the necessary funds.[8] Still others may have had difficulty making the decision. Most late abortions are performed in a hospital setting. In many cases general anesthetic is used if the abortion is performed with a surgical technique. Recovery periods are generally longer and rates of complications higher than for first-trimester abortions.

Abortion is rarely performed in the third trimester, and then generally because of major defects in the fetus. It will probably take considerable effort to locate an abortion provider who performs third-trimester abortions, and because they are few and scattered, you will very likely have to travel a considerable distance. If your primary physician or gynecologist cannot or will not provide information, you can probably get it from Planned Parenthood or one of the other resource organizations listed in this book.

How It Feels

Many factors enter into the sensations you experience during an abortion. You may be given a sedative, or tranquilizer, which relaxes you. You may have general anesthesia, which puts you completely to sleep (this is somewhat more risky, generally unnecessary, and uncommon). You will probably be given a local anesthetic that is injected inside your vagina on either side of your cervix. The injections are uncomfortable, but not usually very painful. After the local anesthetic takes effect, you can feel pulling and pressure, but not pain.

Learning the Skill of Relaxation

Your ability to relax has a lot to do with the discomfort you experience. Anxiety causes your muscles, both generally and in the genital area, to tense up. Muscle tension can cause pain. In addition, tense abdominal and genital muscles make it more difficult for the physician to examine you and to perform the abortion. Relaxation is a skill that requires instruction and practice. If someone tells you to "just relax" in a situation in which it is difficult, or seems critical because you are so tense, tell that person that you are having a hard time and could use some specific suggestions.

Here are some relaxation techniques that you can practice before and during an abortion, dental work, or any other medical procedure. One is imagery. Imagine a relaxing situation that you have enjoyed in the past. We can use the beach as an example (but choose another if the beach isn't pleasant or relaxing for you). Imagine yourself on a beautiful afternoon at the beach, with no one and nothing to worry about. Imagine sensations for each of your senses. Feel the terrycloth of your beach towel against your skin, and notice the sand shifting under the towel as you move and the sand against your toes as they reach past the towel. Smell the sea air and the suntan lotion. Listen to the seagulls and the lapping of the waves. Feel the warmth of the sun on your skin. Look at the shoreline, the birds, the sand castles, the puffy clouds.

Another relaxation technique involves deliberately tensing and then relaxing one muscle group after another. Often we tense our muscles without realizing it. Performing this relaxation exercise helps you to recognize when you are tensing up and allows you to relax muscle groups when you want or need to. Sometimes when you are having a medical procedure, it is helpful to clench muscles in another area of the body. This maneuver distracts you from whatever manipulation or discomfort is associated with the procedure and may help you to relax that area by focusing the tension elsewhere. It's best to try this on yourself; make sure you don't just tense from head to toe. If you are able to relax your vaginal opening, the insertion of the speculum should not be painful.

Controlled breathing is also helpful for relaxation. We rarely notice our own breathing, but we can pay attention to it when we wish to. Notice your breathing pattern. Be sure that you do not hold your breath. Take slow and deep breaths in through your nose and out through your mouth. Think of blowing muscle tension out with each breath. Do not allow yourself to pant, overbreathe, or hyperventilate. Keep the breathing at a slow, steady pace.

There is seldom any reason a woman should be made to feel actual pain during an abortion. You can discuss your preferences and the usual practices of your doctor, clinic, or hospital beforehand. Ask what you should expect to feel and when. Tell them you want to know what is going to happen at each step. Ask what you should do if you feel any pain.

Complications

The complications of abortion fall into several categories. Before an abortion is performed, it must be clear that the pregnancy is actually inside the uterus. Sometimes a pregnancy lodges outside the uterus, most commonly in the fallopian tube—which connects the uterus to the ovary—rather than in the uterus. A tubal, or "ectopic," pregnancy may produce the same symptoms and test results as a normal pregnancy, so the diagnosis may be missed at first. A tubal pregnancy cannot proceed normally because the fallopian tube cannot expand enough to allow the pregnancy to develop. Without medical intervention, the tube may rupture, which is a medical emergency. Ectopic pregnancy is not a complication of abortion, but if it is not diagnosed, it can lead to an unnecessary operation on the uterus. None of the usual abortion techniques will remove a tubal pregnancy. It can be removed either surgically or with medications.

In about 1 out of every 1,000 abortions, the uterus, cervix, or another nearby organ (such as the bladder or bowel) is damaged by the instruments used during the procedure.[3] The damage sometimes heals by itself and sometimes must be surgically repaired. Although vaginal bleeding is normal after abortion, just as during a menstrual period or after childbirth, in rare cases there is excessive bleeding, or hemorrhage, that requires a blood transfusion. Another possible complication is infection introduced into the uterus from the cervix or vagina during the abortion. Antibiotics may be used to prevent infection or to cure it after it has occurred. Finally, the abortion procedure may fail to remove all the tissues of the pregnancy. This situation is called an "incomplete abortion." An incomplete abortion may lead to hemorrhage or to infection of the retained tissue. The treatment of an incomplete abortion consists of a second curettage, by means of suction or scraping, to remove the remaining tissue.

Recovery

After an abortion, you should spend an hour or more resting under nursing observation at the medical facility where the abortion was performed. In most cases, you can return to your usual activities as soon as you feel able. You can expect to experience some cramping and soreness for a couple of days and to have light bleeding for as long as 2 weeks. Most women resume their usual menstrual pattern within 4–6 weeks after an abortion. You should be advised about follow-up care and any recommended limitations on activity by the medical staff. If you aren't, ask.

Several symptoms should alert you to the need to contact the physician who performed the abortion:

- Fever of over 100.4°F
- Severe pain in the abdomen, pelvis, or back
- Vaginal discharge with a foul smell
- Vaginal bleeding heavier than a normal menstrual period
- Cramps lasting more than 2 days after the abortion

You will probably be given an appointment for a follow-up examination to ensure that your healing is progressing satisfactorily. You should also be told whom and where to call if any troubling symptoms occur. It is generally best for the same doctors and nurses who performed a procedure to deal with any complications, because they are most familiar with your case and with their own procedures. However, you can go to a local emergency room if you cannot reach the clinic where the abortion was performed.

The vast majority of these complications can be effectively and fully treated. It is exceedingly rare for a woman to suffer any lasting damage from an abortion performed in a licensed facility by a licensed physician. Less than 1% of all women who have abortions have complications serious enough to require hospitalization, and most recover fully. In fact, women giving birth are 100 times more likely to need major abdominal surgery due to complications than are women having abortions.[2] You may have heard that abortion can result in the loss of one's ability to bear children, an increased risk for breast cancer, or in other permanent negative effects. These are medically inaccurate allegations[8,9] made by anti-choice groups in the hope of frightening women who are considering abortion.

Illegal Abortion

Stories of dire consequences of abortion date from the time when abortions were illegal. When a procedure is illicit, a woman has no opportunity to find out about the qualifications of the staff or the facility, and nowhere to turn in the event of complications. Because the abortion must be performed in secrecy, access to excellent equipment is limited and lighting and sanitation may be poor. Counseling is nonexistent.

The practitioner of illicit abortion may be reluctant to administer medications for the relief of pain or anxiety, either because of time pressures or because the woman must be able to run if the police arrive. There is rarely any opportunity—or willingness—to provide information, to consider feelings, or to observe the patient medically after the abortion. It should also be said that, in times and places where legal access to abortion is limited, there are sometimes highly qualified and dedicated practitioners who are willing to risk criminal prosecution in order to provide women with safe, properly performed abortions.

Contraception After Abortion

You can become pregnant again any time after an abortion. You may feel at first that the problem pregnancy, the decision making, and the medical procedure have been such a focus of attention and emotion that you will never have unprotected sexual intercourse again. But people and circumstances change rapidly. Don't expose yourself to the risk of another problem pregnancy. You can discuss contraceptive methods with a counselor, nurse, or physician who is involved with your abortion before leaving the facility.

Contraceptive possibilities include:

- Hormones in the form of birth control pills, contraceptive implants placed under the skin, or injections
- Barrier methods, including male and female condoms, the diaphragm, and the cervical cap
- Spermicides, which kill sperm before they can cause pregnancy, contained in jellies, creams, or vaginal sponges
- Intrauterine devices (IUDs)
- Male or female sterilization, surgical procedures that interrupt the pathways traveled by sperm or egg and result in the permanent end of fertility for either a man or a woman

The best contraceptive method for you depends on your age, your state of health, your lifestyle, the amount of money you can spend, your access to medical care, your sexual relationships, the nature of your sexual activity, and your preferences.

CHAPTER 6

Religion, Ethics, and Values

Decisions about pregnancy force us to weigh conflicting beliefs, needs, and priorities. Some people consider one particular belief absolute: that ending a pregnancy kills a human being and should be outlawed, just like murder. This chapter explains ethical arguments for and against abortion in order to help you decide what you believe and what you want to do. In the end, there is no way to reconcile the belief that abortion is murder with the belief that a woman has a right and responsibility to decide what to do about her pregnancy. This book respects all thoughtful ethical and religious beliefs but favors a woman's rights to act on her personal ethics in deciding what to do about her own pregnancy.

The Questions

Is an embryo a person?

If an embryo is a person, when in pregnancy does it become a person?

What is the definition of "person," or "human being?"

What rights, if any, does an embryo or fetus have?

Do medical or genetic defects in the embryo affect its rights?

Are the embryo's rights affected by the circumstances of its conception?

Who has a right to participate in an abortion decision?

Is abortion a matter of women's rights or freedom?

Is it right to use fetal tissue for medical treatment or experimentation?

What other rights and values are affected by abortion?

The Embryo's Right to Life

When Does a Fertilized Human Egg Become a Human Being?

Some people look to science to solve the problem of deciding when a fertilized egg becomes a human being. They hope that medical studies will reveal the point in gestation at which an embryo becomes "human." Others are convinced that the egg becomes a human being at the moment of fertilization, because the fertilized egg contains the chromosomes that cause it to develop into a particular individual human being. Each of us developed from a fertilized human egg.

The problem with this reasoning is that every fertilized egg does not develop into a human being. That development requires extremely complicated, specific, circumstances that are available only inside the body of the pregnant woman. Anti-abortion posters often show a fetus late in gestation, looking like a baby, floating in a bubble of fluid, with no evidence of the body of the mother it is growing in. A fertilized human egg has never developed into a person in an artificial environment. In the normal course of life, many eggs die or are shed from the body after fertilization.

In addition, each cell in a human body contains that person's chromosomes, yet a heart cell or a skin cell is not a person and cannot develop into a person. Very specific and complex circumstances are also required for each of the cells that constitute a human body to develop into one particular kind of cell—a liver cell, a brain cell, a bone cell. These circumstances are only beginning to be understood. A human embryo, as long as it is implanted inside its mother, is alive. It develops a beating heart, and somewhat later, reflexes that cause it to jerk its limbs away from an object inserted into its mother's uterus. Do these characteristics make it human? Many non-human creatures have hearts and reflexes. Their lives are not protected by our ethics or our laws.

How else do we define a human being? A human being has a human appearance, a human brain, and human behaviors, feelings, and abilities. It is a unique, individual creature whom other people can recognize. When does an embryo have the capacity to think, feel, and suffer like a human being? These abilities develop gradually, but research into the growth of the human brain indicates that they probably do not occur until relatively late in pregnancy, much later than the vast majority of abortions take place.

Philosophers and religious authorities have pondered the question of when an embryo becomes human for centuries. Often they have equated being human with having a soul. The ancient Greeks believed that this occurred 40 days after conception for a male embryo and 80 days after conception for a female embryo. In European society in the past, the embryo was considered to have a soul when the mother-to-be could feel its movements inside her. This point is called "quickening." Like Aristotle in ancient Greece, the Roman Catholic church, from the 12th to the 19th century, considered the male embryo to have a soul as of 40 days of gestation, and the female embryo only after 80 days. Abortion was permitted prior to the time of "ensoulment."[1]

In the modern-day Roman Catholic church, artificial contraception, many reproductive technologies, and abortion are forbidden. In 1869, the Pope decreed that the Virgin Mary, the mother of Jesus, had been without sin from the time of her conception (the immaculate conception), and that therefore the embryo was a person from the time of conception. Abortion was therefore a sin worthy of excommunication. Despite this decree, there is today an organization called Catholics for a Free Choice, which advocates against the official Church doctrine.[2]

Aside from Roman Catholicism and fundamentalist Christianity, most of the religions widely practiced in the United States permit abortion. In fact, leaders of some religious groups have accused anti-abortion religious groups of violating the U.S. Constitution's required separation of church and state. The Religious Coalition for Reproductive Choice includes representatives of many Protestant Christian and Jewish denominations, as well as Unitarian Universalists, all of whom support reproductive freedom and choice for women.

The Jewish religion consists of several subgroups, the largest of which are Orthodox, Conservative, and Reform. Conservative and Reform Jews believe that abortion is a decision that should be left to the pregnant woman. Orthodox Judaism permits abortion for the first month of pregnancy and frowns upon it after that time. However, abortion is always permitted if the pregnancy threatens the mother's life.[3]

In the Moslem faith, the embryo is considered a person beginning 14 days after conception. Moslems, their religious leaders, and their countries have interpreted this belief in a variety of ways; some permit abortion, some have restrictions, and some forbid it. In practice, most modern Islamic societies forbid abortion after the point at which the embryo is thought to acquire a soul—anywhere from 40 to 120 days.[4]

In the Hindu tradition, classical religious texts dating back to 1500 B.C. express the belief that the fetus has a soul and is human and that abortion is a sin equal to murder.[5] Over time, however, abortion has been treated less and less severely in Hindu society. For instance, in 200 B.C. the Hindu lawgiver Manu treated abortion as little more than a misdemeanor.[4] Today, the abortion rate is very high among Hindus in India, and abortion is viewed as a "necessary evil."[4] The primary reason for abortion in India is sex selection. For both economic and religious reasons, Hindus have a strong preference for sons, and the vast majority of abortions involve female fetuses.

The position of the Greek Orthodox Church on abortion and contraception is very similar to that of the Roman Catholic Church. The official belief of the Greek Orthodox Church is that the fetus is a human being entitled to life. In 1937, Greek Orthodox Archbishop Chrysostomos issued a circular letter condemning both contraception and abortion as threats to family life and evil acts against God's will. However, in the Greek Orthodox tradition, abortion is permitted to save a woman's life.[6]

After all is said and done, the rights of the embryo or fetus are essentially a matter of religious and personal belief, and perhaps more importantly, of personal feelings. Science cannot help. The embryo and fetus cannot express their experiences to us, and none of us remembers our experiences before birth. Our human consciousness does not develop sufficiently to understand specific experiences and record them in memory until several years of age.

Exceptions to Prohibitions on Abortion: Do They Make Sense?

Rape and Incest

Many people opposed to abortion think that abortion is acceptable when a pregnancy resulted from rape or incest. But why should this make a difference if abortion takes the life of a human being? When a child conceived by incest or rape is actually born, it receives all the protection of the law. If other fetuses are be protected, why should these be excluded?

The rationale for laws allowing abortion in cases of incest and rape rests on the concept that no woman, of whatever age, should be required to continue a pregnancy that was begun under these circumstances. This argument ignores the embryo or fetus and any right it may have to develop and be born. It focuses instead on the guilt of the pregnant woman. It assumes that women who are not the victims of rape or incest have complete control over their sexual and contraceptive behavior. If a woman is not forced into the sexual act that makes her pregnant, she should bear the responsibility, and the child.

This attitude puts all the responsibility for sex and conception on women. It implies that women who are virtuous do not experience problem pregnancies, and it seems to make the baby a punishment for a woman's sexual life. However, contraceptive techniques are not foolproof, even when used as prescribed. Some people cannot obtain contraceptive care or afford contraceptive medicines and techniques. Some young people are not provided with enough information about sexuality and reproduction to make responsible choices. Some women are physically, psychologically, and/or financially coerced into sexual activity. The man who has equal ethical and biological responsibility does not have to carry the pregnancy and may not care for the child physically or financially after it is born.

Fetal Defects

There is another fairly common exception to bans on abortion: fetal defects. Many laws and regulations allow abortion when a serious fetal anomaly has been diagnosed before birth. A debate has developed on this question as well: What constitutes a defect? How severe must the defect be to justify an abortion? Who decides whether a given defect warrants termination of the pregnancy?

The numbers and kinds of defects that can be diagnosed before birth continue to grow. There are many variations among human beings. "Normal" is nothing more than an average, and the definition of the point where normal becomes abnormal is a more or less arbitrary statistic.

"Abnormal" is also a matter of the experiences and expectations of the people involved. A condition that some parents would gladly accept might be unbearable to others. A condition that is manageable in some circumstances might be an impossible burden in others. Services and supports for families of children with special needs are limited, and frequent moves, the divorce rate, and the increased numbers of women in the paid work force have diminished the availability of family members to provide care for these children. How should laws or medical professionals decide what burdens to force individuals to undertake and which deviations from normality are too trivial to justify ending a pregnancy?

Some people feel that prospective parents have no right to continue a pregnancy when their child's defects will burden society. Genetics experts worry that their growing ability to identify genetic abnormalities prenatally will result in pressure on pregnant women to have abortions, even if they would prefer not to. One form of pressure might be refusal of medical insurance for a child whose defect was identified before birth.

It is difficult to specify which genetic changes should disqualify a fetus from being born. Many disabled individuals lead gratifying and productive lives. Some of them feel that disabilities like theirs should not be grounds for abortion, whereas others are advocates of individual choice. There is also a concern that using abortion to eliminate "defective" potential people may lead the way to letting or helping disabled, sick, or elderly people die.

Selection of Fetal Characteristics

At the opposite end of the spectrum from abortion for severe disabilities, there is concern that prospective parents will use prenatal diagnostic information to pick and choose characteristics they would like their children to have—hair color, athletic ability—and abort pregnancies that don't fulfill their wishes. The use of abortion to select the sexes of children born into a family is already a possibility and, in some societies, a reality.[4]

Families carrying a sex-linked genetic disease may decide to abort embryos of the involved sex. Families with a strong religious tradition requiring one or more heirs of a given sex (almost always male), and families wishing to balance their families between boys and girls, may also decide to abort some pregnancies on the basis of sex. Geneticists differ among themselves as to whether to give pregnant women information about fetal sex, unless there is suspicion of a sex-linked disease. Some argue that termination of a pregnancy for gender alone is sexist, trivializes the miracle of reproduction, and leaves the pregnant woman vulnerable to family pressures to maintain or terminate her pregnancy. Others argue that the information belongs, philosophically and legally, to the prospective parents. This issue really tests the limits of our comfort with the idea that a woman can make decisions about pregnancy without interference, for any reason important to her.

Who Has a Right to Be Involved in the Decision?

What about family members and the man involved in the pregnancy? Relationships among family members, their responsibilities toward and rights over each other, differ widely among societies. As a society, we have rejected the idea that her sexual partner should have control over a woman's decision. He may be absent or abusive. But he also may have deep and sincere feelings about the decision.

Here is an extreme case example:

> A young man and woman are married. Both are pursuing extremely demanding educations and have high ambitions. They have agreed not to have children for at least 10 years. No woman with children has ever been allowed into the training program the wife has her heart set on. Nevertheless, there is a contraceptive failure, and the wife becomes pregnant. During the time it takes for the pregnancy to be diagnosed and to arrange for an abortion, the husband develops a case of mumps. His testicles are extremely swollen and sore, indicating a high likelihood that they are infected with the virus. He will probably not be able to father biological children after he recovers. He begs his wife to cancel the abortion. He promises he will delay his career progress in order to give parental attention to the baby.

While the potential father's wishes do not have legal weight, that does not mean that they don't have moral and emotional weight.

Potential Grandparents

Potential grandparents also have a major emotional and biological stake in the outcome of a pregnancy. Depending on the culture, particular social group, and individual family, the older generation may have the authority to dictate what the potential parents do, may influence them, or may have nothing to do with the decision. In some societies, parents of married children dictate many aspects of those children's lives. Marriages are made with the express purpose of producing grandchildren.

Mainstream American society tends to frown on this degree of parental involvement in a couple's reproductive life. But our society also incorporates many subcultures that proudly keep other traditions. Although the laws and majority practice do not support a deciding role for potential grandparents, bonds of emotion and tradition with parents play an important part in many women's decisions about their pregnancies. At one extreme, the knowledge that her parents would be profoundly humiliated and alienated by a pregnancy may increase the likelihood that a woman will choose an abortion. At the other extreme is the influence of some parents who regard abortion as immoral or genocidal and who welcome all new babies into the family with warmth and with active participation in child care.

A Case Example

The following case illustrates some of the legitimate, passionate interests that potential grandparents have in a pregnancy.

Two couples come separately to the United States as refugees after all other members of their families are murdered in a war of genocide. Grieving deeply, but determined to build new lives, they work very hard to give their children many advantages that circumstances did not permit them to enjoy. They are comforted by the idea that the cherished values and traditions of their absent relatives will be recreated by the new families they will establish. They imagine little grandchildren looking like their own murdered parents and named after them. One couple has a daughter and one a son. Their children grow up, meet, fall in love, and marry. When the young bride conceives, she and her new husband inform their parents that they have decided to terminate the pregnancy because children would interfere with their lifestyle, and they have decided never to have any. They dismiss the parent's offers of support, memories of lost relatives, and protestations about family tradition, declaring "You're in America now."

Children

A major factor in women's decisions about their pregnancies is their children. They may be thinking about children they plan to have in the future or children they already have. Children already in the family may range in age from young infants to adults. Women feel deeply about providing nurturing circumstances for the lives of their children. They may feel it is their responsibility to see that any children they decide to raise have a father living in the home, a mother who can adapt her schedule to theirs, rooms of their own, or music lessons. Sadly, in many cases, pregnant women have to worry whether their children will have enough to eat, clothing to wear, and someplace decent to live. On the other hand, a woman may feel that a pregnancy is the will of God, and that God will provide for her child.

Abortion and Attitudes Toward Women

Abortion is sometimes viewed as a procedure that liberates women from their traditional roles and allows them to enjoy sexual behavior without fear of pregnancy, to fulfill their own dreams and realize their own, individual ambitions. But abortion is simply a procedure that terminates a pregnancy. Like any other procedure, it can be either liberating or confining, depending on the circumstances.

Abortion can be forced on a woman by circumstances. A woman who wishes to continue a pregnancy can be pressured to have an abortion. Her pregnancy may be an embarrassment to family members. Her sexual partner may be unwilling to make a commitment to the relationship or to a child. Her husband may threaten to abandon the family, leaving his existing children without adequate support, if his wife bears another child. The fact that abortion is available may give her sexual partner an excuse to refuse contraception. In all of these real-life situations, the availability of abortion may actually decrease a woman's ability to do what she would prefer.

Denying access to abortion can also be a way to control or dominate a woman. The inability to end a pregnancy can force a woman to remain in a relationship she would prefer to end. It can remind her of a sexual relationship that was abusive. For example, her parents may want her to suffer because she refused to end a relationship of which they disapproved and because she engaged in sex against their wishes.

Social Attitudes Toward Abortion

Societies shape religious and ethical beliefs and practices. Social attitudes toward abortion are complicated and contradictory. When opinion polls are administered to random members of the population, the answers they give depend on the way the questions are phrased.[7-9] Many people oppose "abortion on demand," but also oppose "governmental interference" in abortion decisions made by a woman and her doctor.

It is not that people are hypocritical, self-deluding, or too careless to reconcile conflicting ideas. They are deeply ambivalent. Differently worded questions resonate with different aspects of our sympathies and sensitivities. Some people have trouble with the idea that a woman could terminate her pregnancy without the need for explanation or approval. But they may have equal difficulty with the idea that the state could intrude into the doctor-patient relationship to supervise, interfere with, and even prevent a medical decision and medical care.

Public sentiment about abortion varies with the stage of pregnancy. Many people who are supportive of free access to abortion during the first weeks of pregnancy have difficulty with the idea of abortion close to delivery. Some people find it helpful to differentiate between a fetus that is entirely dependent on its mother for its continued life, growth, and development and one that is sufficiently developed to survive outside the uterus if prematurely delivered. There is some point during gestation, even if we cannot reach consensus on what that point is, when the concept of the "fetus" merges into the concept of the "unborn child." Some people argue that a woman's right to make decisions about her own body should prevail throughout pregnancy.

Forced Obstetric Interventions

Another important philosophical issue is closely related to the concept of fetus as human being. If the fetus, entirely dependent on its mother for its survival and development into an independent person, is given the full rights of a citizen, there arises the question of whether a woman can be forced, against her will, to undergo treatments that intrude upon her body in the interests of the fetus. The ever-increasing array of diagnostic and therapeutic interventions that can be performed on a fetus within its mother's uterus bring this question into the public eye more and more frequently.

Our laws do not permit any medical intrusion, no matter how minor, on one person's body for the benefit, no matter how great, of another person. No person can be forced to donate one drop of blood to another, even to save the other's life. But the state of pregnancy affects many people's feelings about this prohibition. As a society, we have very powerful feelings about, and expectations of, mothers. The idea of a mother, or mother-to-be, who is not willing to make a physical sacrifice for her child arouses great resentment. The philosophies and emotions that drive these decisions are relevant to abortion. Whose rights should prevail—those of the fetus or those of the mother?

The Medical Uses of Fetal Tissue

The rights of society over the fetus also come up in the area of fetal tissue research. Embryonic and fetal tissue that is aborted, either spontaneously or medically, is extremely useful for the study of the development of the human organism. Treatments for several severe medical illnesses currently depend on human fetal tissue. Some women and some medical scientists are grateful that fetal tissue that is not going to develop into a living person can be utilized for the benefit of other people.

Other groups feel that the use of fetal tissue does not accord the aborted embryo the respect it deserves as a human being in its own right. Some have even voiced the concern that children will be deliberately conceived and then aborted in order to provide a continuing source of tissue. There is no evidence that this has ever actually happened.

Fairness

Limitations on abortion result in gross social inequities. Well-off women and their families are able to obtain safe abortion services, either by getting around the restrictions or by traveling to an area with fewer restrictions. Disadvantaged women are the only ones who truly are affected by the restrictions.

Privacy

Laws allowing abortion only when a pregnancy was caused by rape or incest also force the woman to reveal those painful, intimate circumstances in order to receive medical care, that is, abortion. It is unacceptably intrusive and ultimately impossible for medical care providers or governmental authorities to determine the conditions under which a conception occurred. The attempt to make such a determination prolongs the unwanted pregnancy and delays the abortion. Such laws prevent a woman from making a personal choice as to when, how, and to whom she confides those aspects of her history, and they may expose her to complications and retribution that might not otherwise have occurred. Limitations on abortion also permit or require the government to monitor medical interactions and medical procedures to ensure that no forbidden abortions take place.

In Closing

There is no way to reconcile the position that abortion is the murder of a human being with the position that abortion is the exercise of a woman's right to control what happens in her own body. The current patchwork of laws and practices is the result of hundreds and thousands of local clashes over priorities, values, customs, and religious beliefs. Social and political forces shape the development of official practices and regulations. Meanwhile, individual pregnant women search their own consciences, evaluate their own situations, consider the needs of the people they care about, determine their options, and make the best decisions they can.

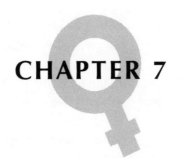

CHAPTER 7

Making the Decision

When you find yourself in an unexpected and difficult situation, it is hard to think clearly. The risks and disadvantages of each possible choice echo in your mind. The benefits of each possible choice bring hopes and wishes to mind. You are tempted to make a decision, act on it, and get it over with, but you are also tempted to postpone the painful decision indefinitely. You may long to share your feelings with people who care about you. You may agonize over whom to tell, realizing that a confidence can never be taken back and may come back to haunt you. You may realize that you don't know as much as you need to know about the position of your religious group, the attitudes of people close to you, the law, or the abortion procedure. The information you want isn't always available and may not register or stay in your memory.

As a result of all this uncertainty, anxieties may interfere with your sleep, your responsibilities, and your relationships, adding new complications to an already demanding situation. And as all this happens, the hours and days of your pregnancy are ticking away. The suggestions in this chapter need not lengthen the process of making your decision, but they can organize and clarify it. There are no perfect answers, but you can make a better decision if you ask yourself the right questions.

You may be reading this book because you or someone close to you made a decision to have, or not to have, an abortion in the past. Although hindsight may be clearer, and sometimes more painful, than foresight, it doesn't capture the emotional reality of a stressful situation. It may be useful, even now, to read and think through some of the material in this chapter. It is never too late to put things in a different perspective. You may find that the reading evokes powerful feelings. You may reexperience your anxiety, your grief, or your disappointment in people who did not behave as you had hoped or expected.

This is not necessarily a bad thing. Give yourself mental and emotional room for your feelings. Realize that no major decision is perfect or made under perfect circumstances. Remember that you did the best you could at the time. Do not blame your reactions entirely on your decision. There were relationships, conflicting values, and other stresses. If you are overcome with feelings you don't think you can handle, if your feelings are interfering with your functioning, or if you just want some help in sorting it all out, make arrangements to see a mental health professional—a psychiatrist, psychologist, social worker, counselor, or religious adviser—who is familiar and comfortable with reproductive decisions. If you don't know where to look, ask your family doctor, religious leader, or the facility where your abortion or delivery was performed.

Assessing Your Situation

Your Background

We are all, to a greater or lesser degree, products of our upbringing. You are born with some personality traits and physical traits. You may have started as a shy or an outgoing person—as a person who loves new and exciting experiences or one who prefers calm, continuity, and familiarity. Then you grew up in one or more families, and the values and experiences of your families shaped your developing attributes into the you who is coping with your current situation.

We all make assumptions, such as: "If I just follow the rules, things will turn out well for me," "Other people will trick you if they can," and "Things just happen to people like me. We can't hope to control them." It's helpful in a difficult situation to review those assumptions, which we may not even realize we make. Some give meaning and structure to our lives. Others, which we picked up along the way, no longer serve any useful purpose and even get in our way. When we examine them, we realize we don't really believe them any more. Here are helpful questions to ask yourself:

How did your family, and other people important to you, feel about sex, conception, contraception, birth, and abortion? Their feelings may not have been exactly the same as the ideas they specifically taught you. For example, parents who were themselves raised to be embarrassed and secretive about sex may try to create a different atmosphere for their children by giving them accurate explanations of sexual body parts and sexual activities. Nevertheless, their discomfort shows. Anecdotes at the dinner table, secrets whispered and overheard, or tones of voice may convey very different messages than the ones the parents think they are communicating to their children.

For example, parents may say that birth is a beautiful thing, but tell terrifying stories about real birth experiences. They may say that both men and women should restrict sex to marriage, but have very different attitudes toward their sons' and their daughters' sexual behavior. They may say that mothers and fathers should share parenting responsibilities, but in practice may leave one parent with the bulk of the responsibility. Try to remember both the words and the feelings that were communicated to you as you developed your own understanding of sexuality, reproduction, and parenthood, because they are influencing you now.

In addition to the teachings and attitudes passed along in families, religions, and schools are the experiences people actually have. In the course of your life, you have known pregnant women, women who have new babies, and perhaps women who have had abortions. Your mother gave birth to you. You have made your own observations about the effects of pregnancy, motherhood, and abortion on women and their lives and families. After making individual observations, especially early in life, we tend to generalize them to other situations. For example, many children feel displaced when their mothers become pregnant and give birth to new babies. They may grow into women who associate pregnancy and childbirth with loneliness or separation. This expectation can instill fear in a woman making a decision about a pregnancy. On the other hand, the birth of a new baby can be a time of joy. Memories of family togetherness—or problems—can arouse expectations that may or may not be appropriate to your current situation.

Lastly, you may have had your own past experiences of pregnancy, abortion, birth, or mothering. They will certainly give you important information about your reactions, your interests, your capabilities, and your preferences. They will probably have more influence on your decision than any other factor. If you have had negative experiences and you are reluctant to make the same decisions again, you may want to reflect whether the bad aspects of the past experiences could be corrected the next time around. You were younger when the past experience occurred. Other people may have dominated your decision. You may not have been able to choose your care providers or to express your concerns and preferences. You may now have different people to turn to for advice and support. On the other hand, things may not have changed. You may have false hopes of replacing a bad experience.

Your Personal Circumstances

The next step in thinking through your decision is to assess your own current situation. Many people focus first on money. Can you afford to have a baby? Having a child may decrease your ability to earn money by disrupting and delaying your education and your career advancement. This is particularly true if you are a teenager, and more so if the baby is not your first.

There are no rules about the amount of money you need. There are magazine articles counting the hundreds of thousands of dollars people spend on obstetric care, baby furniture and supplies, children's clothing, music lessons, and college educations. Other people get by happily and successfully with a few hand-me-downs and public schools. Only you can know what's important to you. There is a difference between deciding to manage parenthood on a shoestring and denying the reality of the cost of basic necessities like health care, food, and shelter. A certain amount of money does make things easier.

You may be concerned about finding the money to pay for a medical examination, childbirth, or an abortion. If you think you may want to deliver the baby and allow him or her to be adopted, the adopting parents or adoption agency may help you with the expenses of pregnancy and delivery. Your health insurance may cover some or all of your expenses; you will probably need to call the insurance office to get the information you need. But you may not want the insurance office (at work, school, or the insurance company itself), or your employer or your co-workers, to know that you are pregnant and considering an abortion. You may be able to find someone to ask for you. You may ask the insurance office for a written promise that your question will be kept in confidence. This can be a real problem, and there is not always an acceptable answer.

Related to money is the question of a place to live. This is mainly a concern for women who plan to continue their pregnancies. Can you, and do you wish to, remain in your current living situation after having an abortion or a baby? Is it big, convenient, and safe enough? How would the other people living with you, if any, react to your decision? Are there people to help you? Are there other alternatives, and what are the answers to the same questions about them?

What is the state of your physical and mental health? Have you had medical or psychiatric problems in the past? How serious were they? What brought them on, and what helped to resolve them? If you have ongoing medical or psychiatric problems, you will want to think about how a pregnancy or an abortion is likely to affect them. Medications or other treatments you are taking must be taken into consideration in the management of your pregnancy and your delivery or abortion. Are you well enough to assume parental responsibilities? If you are under the care of a health professional, you will want to discuss these questions with that person as soon as possible. If you are not currently in care, this is a good time for an evaluation. Consultation with a subspecialist expert may be helpful.

If you have any concerns about confidentiality, make that clear before you explain your problem, and do not proceed until you have received assurances that your concerns will not be shared with anyone. Confidentiality in medical communications is required by ethical codes and by law, but lapses can still occur, particularly if the health care provider works with more than one member of a family or couple or reports to an institution such as a corporation, the military, or the justice system. You may want to seek consultation outside your system.

Your Family

In the Western world, some people live their whole lives in the bosoms of their families, some

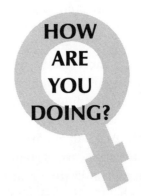

HOW ARE YOU DOING?

Are you forgetting meals or having trouble eating more than a few bites? Are you stuffing yourself and feeling bad about it?

Is worrying about your decision making it difficult to fall asleep or stay asleep? Do you try to escape by sleeping more than usual?

Are you finding it hard to concentrate all the way through a task or pay attention all the way through a conversation, television program, movie, or newspaper story?

Has the pleasure gone out of things you usually enjoy?

Do you avoid spending time with people whose company you used to like?

Are you more irritable or angry than usual? (You may have good reason to be.) Are you crabbier than you would like with people you care about?

Are you preoccupied with sad, pessimistic thoughts and feelings? Do you find yourself crying once or more every day?

Again, you may have good reason to feel that way, but it is important to assess whether the concern over your pregnancy has cast a pall over everything in your life, even things that usually make you feel happy and hopeful.

Does your mood change suddenly for no obvious reason?

Do you find yourself generally nervous, jumpy, and worried about things in general or nothing in particular?

Are you feeling overly guilty?

Are you experiencing physical symptoms like stomach aches, headaches, upset stomach, or others not directly caused by pregnancy?

These symptoms are an indication that you should consider seeing your doctor, religious adviser, or a mental health professional—a counselor, social worker, psychologist, or psychiatrist. You may have a clinical depression or anxiety disorder. These illnesses are very common and very treatable.

If you are experiencing mild symptoms that don't interfere with your functioning, give yourself room for them. There may be simple things you can do to help yourself feel better: eat nutritious and comforting meals, take a warm bath, go for a walk, call a friend, remind yourself that millions and millions of women have found themselves in the same situation.

leave their families at an early age and keep their distance, and most are somewhere between these two extremes. Are you close to family members? How would they feel about the alternatives you are considering? Do they have the time, energy, and other resources to help you?

In addition to your family of origin, in which you are a daughter, a sister, a cousin, or other relative, you have a family or relationship in which you are the parent or potential parent. If you have children, you will consider their number, their ages, and any special problems or needs they have.

Do you just want a baby? Some women have trouble adjusting to the changing needs of children as they become increasingly independent. Any child you have will be a baby for a short time and will be a child, adolescent, and adult for a much longer time. Other women dread caring for an infant and endure it only in order to watch the baby develop into an active child and adult. There is so much social pressure on women to enjoy motherhood that it is hard to know how people really feel.

There are no hard-and-fast rules about how many years should separate the children in a family. What matters most is the parents' preferences and their ability to deal with the family they choose to have. Meeting the needs of two babies less than 18 months apart is demanding. It is not fair to expect the older baby to behave like a big boy or girl simply because another child is born. Two babies can be fun, and can grow up to be best friends, or can be a nightmare and resent each other. A child born long after one or more other siblings will disrupt the family lifestyle all over again. He or she will probably not enjoy a playmate relationship with his or her siblings but may enjoy looking up to them and learning from them. It is not so much a matter of the rooms in your house as the room in your life and your heart.

The man with whom your pregnancy was begun may or may not be your legal husband (you may even have a different legal husband). He is a central character in your situation. That is true even if you don't know where he is and don't expect to see him ever again. He is a focus because your decision and your feelings about your pregnancy can never be entirely separate from your relationship with him. It is especially difficult, but not uncommon, to have to make a decision about a pregnancy in the midst of grief over the end of a relationship or uncertainty about its future. Problems with relationships are a major reason pregnancies become problem pregnancies. Is your relationship going to be a help or a hindrance as you make your decision?

If the man is a part of your current life, you probably care more about his preferences and feelings than about anyone else's. He may be upset about his role in the situation and uncertain about what decision is best, or he may have a strong opinion one way or the other. He may recognize the fact that the decision is ultimately yours and offer to support whichever decision you make, or he may make his support contingent upon your following his preference. You may not be sure that he is realistic or dependable. Most likely, he will behave in the future more or less as he has in the past.

Domestic Violence: A Special Case

A relationship with a man who is violent is dangerous. You may assume or hope that your pregnancy will bring you closer together, that he will now protect and nurture you. Unfortunately, you are probably mistaken. Domestic violence actually often increases during pregnancy.[1] Domestic violence often occurs in a cyclical pattern. Gradually increasing tension is finally broken by an episode of violence, followed by apologies, affection, and promises before the tension building begins all over again.

Many women who are physically abused try to push the violent episodes out of their minds after they occur. They blame themselves for their partners' violence. They feel ashamed and alone. Many women think that domestic violence only occurs in poor families or among criminals. Actually, violence between domestic partners occurs in every social and economic class.

A problem pregnancy can be an opportunity to look clearly at your relationship and take steps to protect yourself. Many states and cities have hotline telephone numbers listed in the telephone directory, on public buses and trains, in medical offices, on grocery store bulletin boards, and in other public places so that abused women can obtain help in privacy. The police are increasingly aware of the frequency and dangers of domestic violence. Lastly, there are shelters where abused women and their children can live for a time in safety, learn about community resources, and consider their options. The "Resources" section at the end of this book contains more information about potential resources for women who find themselves in a violent situation and are looking for help.

Your Coping Style

In the midst of a difficult situation, you can forget to eat, to sleep, to relax. If you have not decided to tell people close to you that you are in the midst of making a decision about a pregnancy, they may misunderstand or ignore any signs of your distress. They may think it best to leave you alone, urge you to get some rest, or try to tempt you with invitations to have fun. You may even try to convince them that nothing is bothering you.

There is no evidence that women faced with problem pregnancies cannot make careful, sensible choices among their options. They can and they do. However, there may be times when it doesn't feel that way.

What is your usual style of coping with demanding situations? You probably take it for granted and never think about it. Some people seek out all their friends and relatives, share their problem, and ask for advice and support. Do these conversations make you feel better or worse? Other people withdraw to think, calm down, and regroup. Think about whether your time alone is helping you or leaving you feeling more upset and lonely. Some people seek a friend, a person who has gone through the same experience, or a professional expert to advise them about what to do and then follow that advice. Others want lots of information so that they can make their own decisions. (The fact that you are reading this book may mean that this is your style.)

Some people show and feel little emotion during a crisis but collapse after it is over. Other people act and feel overwhelmed, convinced they will never get through it, but come through. Some people have to put aside some of their usual responsibilities to make mental and emotional space to consider their options; others throw themselves into their work or other activities to distract themselves. No one of these coping styles is right or wrong. It's only a matter of what works for each individual. Acknowledging what you usually do may help you to recognize that the things you are doing and feeling now are your usual style, the style that always helps you get through the crisis in the end. On the other hand, you may notice that, for some reason, your usual style isn't helpful. Try something new.

Organizing a Support System

Who, outside your family, is important to you? Your social support system includes individual people and institutions like your religion, your employer or school, and public and private social service agencies such as Public Assistance and Children and Family Services. Your need for outside support will depend on your personal style and your life plans. Many of the concerns about families apply to friends and other social contacts as well. Think about who is likely to be there for you, and whom you want to be there, as you make and live with this decision.

Who Might Help, and How Will They React?

Think about all the people you could talk to. For each person, recall your past experiences with them. What experiences has this person had with pregnancy, abortion, childbirth, and parenting? What values and religious beliefs does the person have? What will be their personal stake in your decision? For example, will the person expect to help you take care of a child if you have one? Will this be the person to pay for an abortion? Will this news threaten to tie the person to a relationship he would prefer to end, or that he thinks never started? Will he hope to tie you to a relationship you would prefer to end, or think never started? Is this a potential grandparent who has been eagerly hoping to have a grandchild?

Don't set yourself up for a disappointment. Powerful feelings are not always acknowledged, but they are revealed in the ways people behave and the things they say. Relatives and friends may be jealous of your relationship, worried that you will get attention and care because you are pregnant, or concerned that a child you might have would compete for attention with a child of theirs. They may feel that your pregnancy would be an embarrassment, or that people will think badly of the family if they learn you've had an abortion. They may think you are too young, or too old, to have a baby. They may disapprove of the potential baby's father. They may feel that you should be punished because you engaged in sexual activity and became pregnant; the punishment might be either an abortion or pregnancy and childbirth.

How does this person really feel about you? Sometimes people say nice things about another person but behave in a way that undermines and hurts that person. Are there long-standing rivalries and competition? Has the person shown respect for your feelings and preferences?

Deciding What You Want From Others

There are many forms of support. Different people have different expectations, and the differences can result in painful, unexpected clashes. People sometimes withdraw when they hear a powerful piece of news, partly because it stirs up feelings in them and partly because they are concerned that they will be drawn into a situation full of unpredictable or overwhelming demands.

Perhaps you feel that this pregnancy is a terrible piece of bad luck, and what you want a particular person to do is to acknowledge the difficult situation you're in and the pain you're feeling—that is, give you sympathy. Perhaps you have mixed feelings of pride, shock, resentment, hope, or guilt. Some of these feelings may surprise you or make you uneasy. What you want is someone who will understand how you feel and help you to accept them—empathy. Perhaps you just want company. You may want a person to listen, express sympathy or empathy, and then leave you alone to make your decision and get on with your life. Sometimes what you want is more concrete. It may be money, a place to stay for a while, a companion for an afternoon or evening, or someone to go to the doctor's office, clinic, or hospital with you.

People need to know what is being asked of them. This gives you an opportunity to figure out what you want. Then it is

STARTING THE DIALOGUE

Your predictions about people may not be correct. Human beings are complicated, and reproductive decisions can provoke unexpected responses. The very relatives you count on may be jealous, condemning, angry, or unavailable. The people you assume will reject your decision may rise to the occasion when you really need them. Make the best prediction you can and try to take the discussion in small steps.

Here are some examples of ways to start the conversation:

- "Do you have a few minutes when we could talk?"

relatively simple to let the other person know: "I'd appreciate an hour with you so you can tell me what your abortion was like," "I need to borrow $300 for a couple of months," "Would you take care of my children for an afternoon so that I can go to the clinic?" "Can I stay with you until my family cools off?" "Could you just listen and tell me I'll be okay?"

Talking to Children

It is not reasonable to expect children to help you make your decision, but it is reasonable to expect that they will know that something is going on and ask you about it. To understand abortion, a child must be mature enough to understand the concept of an embryo or fetus that the child can't see, that has the potential to become a real baby but that isn't one yet. Explain that a decision to have an abortion doesn't mean you reject parenthood or the children you already have; it may reflect your satisfaction with the family you have. Abortion can be a positive choice. One last consideration with children is the fact that they are very likely to tell other people whatever they know or think.

- "I would like to talk to you about a worry that is on my mind."
- "I want to ask for your understanding and help about something."
- I know you are busy and have a lot on your mind. Please tell me if it is too much for you to hear about one more problem."
- "There is a problem we share, and we need to talk about it together."
- "I really need your help."

Watch and listen to the other person. The person may say that he or she wants to help but show you the contrary by turning away, cutting off the conversation, or telling you how many troubles he or she already has. The person's statements may not be warm, but he or she may show concern and a willingness to help by listening patiently or giving you a reassuring pat.

Confidentiality

How important is it to you that your conversation be confidential? In the real world, you can never be absolutely sure of confidentiality. The most well-meaning people have slips of the tongue. There are extreme circumstances in which a woman feels that her life or her future may be threatened if a certain person learns of her pregnancy or her abortion. If you are in extreme circumstances, you will have to be extremely careful, probably restricting your communications to medical and legal or court personnel who are required by law to observe confidentiality. Under less dangerous circumstances, you have to weigh your need to get advice and support against the chances that information about your pregnancy and decision will reach people you would not have chosen to tell. You may also have to consider whether your request for confidence is an imposition on a particular person. For example, your husband or boyfriend's best friend and immediate family members will probably find it awkward to keep the secret from him.

If you are below legal age, your confidentiality may be limited by law. Some states require that one or both of your parents be notified, or give consent, before you can have an abortion. These laws and regulations do not affect your discussions with a doctor, counselor, or judge before you decide to have an abortion, however. Those conversations are still confidential—but ask the doctor, counselor, or lawyer before you talk, just to make sure.

How to Arrange the Conversation

The circumstances.   Sometimes you can't have much control over the circumstances of a conversation. It may be so difficult to talk about your situation that you have to blurt it out whenever you can muster the courage. Your opportunities to talk to the other person may be limited by your schedules, or they may occur at times that are full of other obligations, like job duties or child care. It would be ideal to have every important conversation in a quiet, private place, without interruptions or limitations of time, but that is rarely possible and may even make people uncomfortable. If you do prefer a quiet time and place, give yourself permission to try to arrange one.

The timing.   Another factor you want to consider is when to tell another person. Your timing will depend to some degree on what you want from the person. If you want sympathy and reassurance at the time of the initial surprise of an unexpected pregnancy, you obviously want to talk to someone right away. If you want information or help thinking through a decision, you can wait a few days. If you will not need help from a particular person until after you have made your decision, because the help you want is in providing company, money, child care, or transportation, you can wait to tell the person a bit longer. Don't rush.

You may want to take into consideration how the person will feel about the timing of your conversation. You may have to explain why you didn't wish this person to participate in the decision itself or why you spoke to one person before another. A person who cares about you needs to understand that you had to think this decision through by yourself or with one or two of the others most closely involved.

The wording.   The words you choose will have a significant influence on how another person reacts. Remember that old story about the man whose car developed a flat tire on a country road? He hoped to borrow a jack at a farmhouse he spotted nearby, but he was very worried that the people who lived there would refuse. As he trudged toward the house, increasingly frustrating scenarios ran through his mind. By the time he knocked on the farmhouse door, he had gotten himself into such a state that he shouted "Keep your stupid jack!"

Even though you may feel upset, think how best to approach this particular individual. Some of our significant others respond to logic, and others to emotions. Some want to be our one special helper, and others are more likely to help if others are already involved. Sometimes it is useful to remind the person of understanding and help you have given in the past, but sometimes it makes the person feel overly pressured.

Preparing yourself for negative responses.   Letting down your guard, asking for help, and then being rejected is an especially painful experience. Remember that decisions about pregnancy are heavily emotionally weighted, and that the other person, no matter how close to you, may well have emotional baggage you don't know about. Your decision and your well-being don't depend on the response of any one person. No other person can make this decision for you or make you feel fine.

Like millions of women before you, you can come through this episode in your life even stronger and wiser than you came into it. If another person's reaction is not just what you hoped, you may feel a tremendous letdown. Don't let yourself overreact. Take a deep breath, end the conversation, find something soothing to do for a little while, and wait to mentally process the interaction later, when you have more distance and perspective.

Getting Information

Individual Medical Care Providers

If you have an ongoing relationship with a physician, midwife, or nurse practitioner whom you like and trust, you may naturally look to that person for information. However, it may be that you are not certain whether you want this person to know about your situation. The person may have negative religious or philosophical beliefs concerning abortion. You may share the care provider with family members or friends and may have concerns about whether it will be realistically possible for the person to keep your situation confidential. You may have reason to feel that the person is not particularly knowledgeable about the information you need. You may not feel comfortable talking to the person, or you may be confident that the person can provide information without trying to influence your decision.

As with a family member or friend, you can have a preliminary conversation without revealing the details of your problem. It is perfectly appropriate to make an appointment just to talk. Tell the person who makes the appointments that is what you want, and that you need an appointment within the next several days. If the receptionist is not helpful, it is often useful to speak directly to the care provider. Tell the receptionist that you are an ongoing patient, that you need to speak to the doctor on the telephone within a day or two, and that you are willing to call at whatever time is convenient for the practitioner. The practitioner can often find time in the schedule when the receptionist can't. You can ask the practitioner whether you can speak about something in complete confidentiality. You can say that you want only information at this point. Then you can get a sense of how the practitioner reacts to you and your situation.

Many people have no regular physician. You could use this occasion to begin a relationship with a family doctor or nurse practitioner, or you might want to see a gynecologist who specializes in women's reproductive health. You may want to obtain information from a provider who provides abortion and/or obstetric services so that you can continue your care with the same person once you reach your decision.

You can obtain a referral to a health care provider from a friend or relative, a local hospital, Planned Parenthood, a medical school, or a physician referral service. You should be aware that a referral service is probably supported by the physicians on its lists. Your choice of health care provider may be limited by your health care insurance or financial circumstances. There is some source of free care in most areas of the country; you can try calling the state medical school gynecology clinic or the city or county hospital. Some institutions supported by public funds will not deal with the subject of abortion at all; ask in advance.

If you have health insurance of some sort, this is a good time to check what it covers. At the time this chapter is being written, the majority of Americans' health insurance covers abortion services. Your health insurance or health maintenance organization may allow you to go directly to the health care provider of your choice, or it may require that you see a generalist nurse or doctor first. Make it clear that what you want is a consultation.

The conversation should be kept confidential; you may want to ask what information will be shared with your employer or any other agency, such as a utilization review company or the government. You may have to sign a form permitting your records to be shared with reviewers. Reviewers have an obligation to keep your medical records confidential, too, but if you are uncomfortable, your only choice may be to pay for the consultation out of your own pocket.

Once you have an appointment with a care provider, think about the information you want. Don't put limitations inside your head on your own thoughts, feelings, and questions. Don't tell yourself that you're childish, demanding, unintelligent, or unsophisticated. You can decide which questions you will actually ask afterwards. Here are questions you might want to ask about abortion. There is more leisure to consider questions about pregnancy, childbirth, and parenting, and there are other good books on those subjects. A list of those resources can be found in a section at the end of this book.

- Where can I get an abortion?
- If there is more than one choice, what are the pros and cons of each one?
- Do I have any medical conditions that might have a bearing on my decision?
- How much does an abortion cost in whichever settings are available to me?
- Can somebody be with me while I have an abortion?

When you arrive for the appointment, make it clear that you are there to get information. This may be an unusual request in the doctor's office or clinic, but it is perfectly legitimate. Don't let anyone make you feel bad about it. If you have not had a physical examination, it is probably a good idea to have one now, both to confirm the pregnancy and to check on your general physical condition. If you have recently had a physical and gynecologic examination, you may not need one at this visit.

In some medical facilities, patients are expected to take off their clothes before seeing the care provider. You may feel more comfortable having your discussion with your clothes on, and you may tell the staff that's what you want to do. Whenever you try to get what you need from a medical setting, you have to balance your needs against the resentment the staff may feel about changing their comfortable routines. After you have your own preferences clear in your mind, you can play it by ear, step by step.

Clinics and Hospitals

Other sources of information about abortion procedures are Planned Parenthood and other family planning clinics, as well as abortion facilities themselves. Abortion clinics vary; some are run for profit and may not present a balanced picture of your choices. It is legitimate to ask about the ownership and funding of the clinic if you want to know. Some physicians perform abortions in their private offices; again, it is helpful to get a referral from a friend or relative who knows the doctor. It is also important to trust your own feelings about the clinic or physician.

Planned Parenthood, which is listed in the telephone book, is a reliable source of information. The same is generally true of medical schools and general hospitals, although some are operated by religious groups opposed to abortion. The religious affiliation is not always apparent from the name of the institution; if you are not sure, ask. In facilities such as these, the staff will probably refuse to discuss abortion.

Advertisements

You may see advertisements offering help for pregnant women—in the telephone directory, on billboards, and on public buses and trains. These advertisements may be misleading. In some cases they will lead you to a group that exists for the sole purpose of preventing women from having abortions. They may tell you that they and the government can assure you of support if you decide to continue your pregnancy and give birth to a baby. They may not be able to fulfill those promises. Some of these groups will attempt to frighten you with misinformation about the process or aftereffects of abortion or with grisly pictures.[2] These experiences can be traumatic, so be wary of these sources of information.

Religious Information

For accurate information on religion and abortion, you can go to a religious institution. You may choose a seminary, a church, a mosque or temple, or the local headquarters of a particular religion. You can find them in the telephone book under the name of the religious faith. The Religious Coalition for Reproductive Rights can provide a comprehensive overview of the beliefs of various religions. There is also an organization called Catholics for Freedom of Choice. The addresses and telephone numbers of both of these organizations are listed in the "Resources" section of this book. These are groups that support women's choices about whether to continue or terminate pregnancies, and in some cases they oppose the positions of their parent religions.

You may wish to obtain information from your own priest, minister, rabbi, or other religious leader. You may have a long-standing, supportive relationship with this individual. You may not feel comfortable with your decision until you know the positions of your religion and your religious leader. At the same time, you will want to consider whether this particular individual has a comprehensive knowledge of your religion's positions on reproduction and whether he or she will be supportive. Religious leaders are human, and variable—they have judgmental feelings, and sometimes they mix those feelings with their religious information. Sometimes a friend or relative or a reproductive health care provider or counselor will be able to recommend another leader in the same faith who is more understanding and/or better informed.

Processing Information

Often, just when you need information the most, it's hardest to register it in your mind and think it through. When you're making an important and emotional decision, you usually need to go over information several times. You may be distracted by the person talking to you and the institutional setting in which you find yourself. You may be preoccupied with the image of yourself having an abortion or cuddling a new baby. Don't expect yourself to take in every bit of information as it is given. Give yourself a few hours, a night's sleep, or a day or two to let it sink in. Write down the important points.

After you've spoken with someone, you may realize that you forgot to ask certain questions and that you have new ones. Contact the original source of information to say that the information was very helpful, that you have been thinking about it, and that there are a couple of issues that you would like to clarify. In fact, you may want to ask at the time of the original conversation whether it would be all right to call in a day or two, after you have had time to digest the information.

Your Decision and Its Outcome

Time Pressures

If you are the kind of person who loses track of time under pressure, it may be helpful to get a calendar in order to track the course of your pregnancy and the steps in the decision-making and outcome process day by day. Plan a course of action, one step at a time, and do something, no matter how small, now and every day. The something may be consulting with a friend, making an appointment to see a religious leader or doctor, picking up information at a family planning clinic, finding a baby-sitter, or making a financial arrangement. Remember that appointments can be canceled and money can be returned. A decision to have an abortion is not final until you decide that it is.

You may be preoccupied with dreams of a close relationship with the man with whom you created your pregnancy. Or you may be angry at him and dream of getting revenge, whether by ending the pregnancy, forcing him to support you and a baby, giving up a baby for adoption, or caring for a baby he doesn't have the privilege of knowing. You may imagine yourself playing pat-a-cake with a rosy-cheeked baby or wiping away a happy tear as a brilliant 18-year-old receives honors at graduation. You may have a mental image of your family during the holidays, doting on you and your beautiful toddler.

Or you may hope that the opportunity to end this pregnancy will allow you to finish your education, get the job of your dreams, make the relationship of your dreams, and live the life you've always wanted. These dreams may not be realistic, but being realistic doesn't have to make you feel bad, either. Being realistic doesn't mean being pessimistic and guilty; it means getting accurate information and using it to make the best decision you can. Most women are satisfied with their own decisions about problem pregnancies.

Now picture yourself in a week, a month, 6 months, a year, 5 years, and 20 years, after having an abortion, having a baby and caring for it, or having a baby and allowing others to take custody of it.

- Where will you be living?
- How will you be supported financially?

- What education will you be about to have, or have had?
- What will be your religious beliefs, affiliations, and practices?
- Who will be the important people in your life, and what will be the nature of those relationships? Will you be in a committed, long-term relationship with one particular person?
- Will you have children, either as a result of this pregnancy or other pregnancies you have already had or would like to have?
- What career will you be looking forward to or pursuing?
- What will be the activities outside of work that you enjoy, and what time and energy will you wish and be able to devote to them?

Human beings can be amazingly adaptable. Human beings also change their minds and feelings over time as they learn and have new experiences. Their beliefs and feelings about a decision may change from relief to regret to acceptance and back again several times during their lives. At the same time, people's basic values and personalities do not easily change. With the help of the careful soul-searching and information-gathering recommended in this book, you, like most women making a decision about abortion, can choose the course of action that will be best for you not only now but throughout your future.

Here is the most important question of all: In the privacy of your own mind, heart, and soul, how will you feel about the decision you are now about to make?

CHAPTER 8

Making the Arrangements

The suggestions in this chapter are gathered here so that you can access the information you need when you have made a decision to have an abortion and are ready to make the arrangements. Some people deal with a medical experience by thinking about it as little as possible. They want to get a recommendation for an abortion clinic from someone they trust, make an appointment, go through the various procedures, and put the experience behind them. Other people want to know and think about it as much as possible. Probably most of the people reading this book like to do things that way. In general, people who experience their anxieties and ask their questions do better emotionally after a medical procedure than those who don't. If your pregnancy is fairly advanced, you may have to compress this process into a few hours or days—but that doesn't mean it can't happen at all.

Choosing the Clinic

Some women don't have a choice of where to have an abortion because of financial limitations, legal restrictions, or travel problems. But sometimes there are options you haven't thought of. This section may help you to find them. Even when you do not have the opportunity to choose among various places, you may be able to use some of the ideas in this section to make your abortion experience as close as possible to what you do want.

To find out where abortions may be obtained in your area, ask a friend or a health professional, the local Planned Parenthood clinic listed in your telephone book, the national Planned Parenthood office, or one of the other organizations listed in the "Resources" section of this book. You can call the clinic and ask for an appointment to see the facility and speak to the staff. Some clinics are open only on certain days of the week or month, and some are careful about visitors for security reasons. Explain your situation and your reasons for wanting the appointment. If the facility is not willing to make such an appointment, ask why not. Perhaps they can answer some of your questions over the telephone. You will get a sense of the staff's attitudes towards patients' needs by their responses to your call.

Decide whether you would be more comfortable closer to or farther from your home, school, work, friends, or relatives, or in one neighborhood rather than another. What are the parking arrangements? Security and freedom from harassment may be considerations. You can ask the clinic whether there have been security problems or demonstrators. If there have been, they may be able to put you in touch with a group of volunteers who accompany women from their cars or other transportation to the clinic entrance. Find out what hours and days they operate. Is there a waiting list, or can they take you as soon as you wish? Clinic personnel may also be able to help you with questions about whether parental notification or consent is required for minors and whether there is a mandatory waiting period.

Some women find it very helpful to visit the clinic and meet the staff beforehand rather than going there for the first time to have the abortion itself. You can observe how the staff behave, how the other patients are treated, and what the physical space looks like. You can ask questions in person. It may be possible to speak with a counselor on this visit.

You should be able to find out exactly what the abortion will cost. Do not hesitate to ask whether the price includes counseling, the examinations and testing required for the abortion, and follow-up care after the abortion. You can ask whether there is a sliding-fee scale for those with financial hardship. You will have to find out whether your health insurance, if you have it, covers abortion. From the clinic, you need to know what documents you will need to bring in order for your health insurance company to pay for the abortion. Will the clinic bill the insurance company, or will they require you to pay and obtain your own reimbursement from the company? If the insurance company pays a part of the expenses, what amount will you need to pay? Will you be expected to bring a check, money order, or cash with you, or will the clinic bill you?

Anesthesia and Other Procedures

You will probably want to know what anesthetic and surgical techniques will be used for the abortion and whether you have any choice. Do you have a strong preference for being awake, asleep, or sedated during the procedure? Each has its advantages and disadvantages. If you are not comfortable with the procedures used by the clinic, even after they have been explained, and there is another procedure you have learned about that you would prefer, you can ask for that procedure. However, you have to balance your preference against the advantages of the staff's experience with the techniques they generally use. If there are other clinic possibilities, you may want to explore them and their techniques instead.

If you do not understand any medical jargon the clinic staff use, ask that it be translated into ordinary English. Most people are overly respectful of medical personnel and hate to ask questions, no matter how appropriate. If you are one of those people, you will have to push yourself to get the information you need. This is a worthwhile experience, not only now, but also for dealing with medical personnel for the rest of your life. Many women who have abortions find that making and carrying out the decision is a turning point in their sense of control over their lives.

Counseling

You may or may not want counseling provided by the clinic. At many facilities, counseling is mandatory. The staff must discuss your decision with you to make sure you are fully informed about your options and the abortion procedure, and that you have made the decision to have the abortion of your own free will. You may discuss your social supports and resources; the reasons for your decision to terminate your pregnancy; and the attitudes and support of your friends, family, and the man with whom the pregnancy was begun. The counselor will also want to get a sense of how you are doing in general.

The counselor should want to understand your circumstances and the basis for your decision to have an abortion. Much of the counseling process will cover the issues in this book. The counselor should not try to influence your decision, except in one circumstance. If the counselor or the abortion provider does not feel you are truly comfortable with your decision, he or she should strongly recommend that you postpone acting upon your decision until you have worked out whatever problems are identified in the counseling session. The facility may refuse to perform the abortion if they feel you cannot make a fully informed decision.

After the abortion, you should be offered information about contraception and a referral for any contraceptive care you wish that is not provided by the clinic. You may be certain that you will never expose yourself to a problem pregnancy again, but you can't rely on that determination to keep pregnancies from happening. Expect to be susceptible to pregnancy the moment the abortion is over, and plan accordingly.

You can also request referral to a mental health professional either before or after the abortion. There should be no stigma attached to this request. The fact that you wish to explore and deal with your feelings, relationships, and coping skills is a sign of strength, not weakness. Remember that several states have passed laws requiring that abortion providers deliver a set speech to women before they have abortions. The constitutionality of these provisions have been upheld by the U.S. Supreme Court. This is not really counseling.

Some Practical Questions

You will want to know how to arrange your schedule for the abortion. Here is a checklist of things to consider:

- When do you need to arrive at the clinic? How long will you have to wait?
- Should you bring something like a magazine, book, or handwork to pass the time?
- Is there anything else, such as sanitary pads, that you should bring along?
- Will there be any laboratory tests that you have to take now or on the day of the abortion? If so, what are they, what do they cost, and how must they be paid for?
- Will you have a general physical examination and/or pelvic (vaginal) examination before the procedure? If so, who will perform them?
- Can you meet the clinic professionals ahead of time?
- How long will the abortion itself take?
- How long will you be in the clinic after the abortion?
- Who will perform the abortion?
- Can a friend or relative be present during the abortion?
- If you have questions during the procedure, whom should you ask?
- What sensations should you expect?
- Whom should you tell if you don't understand what you are feeling or if you feel unexpected pain? What can you expect them to do about it?

You will also want to know about routine follow-up after the abortion:

- Do they expect you to come back for a checkup, and, if so, when?
- What symptoms might you have immediately and in the hours and days after the abortion?

- If you have general anesthesia, what aftereffects should you anticipate?
- If you will have any local anesthesia, when is it likely to wear off?
- Is it necessary for someone to drive you or accompany you home? Can you take public transportation, or will you have to travel in a car?
- Will there be restrictions on your activities after the abortion, and, if so, which ones and for how long? How dangerous will it be if you are not able to follow them?
- When should you count on being able to assume responsibility for your household and being able to return to work or school?
- What are the arrangements for medical care if you have complications such as excess bleeding or an infection?
- What if there are complications during the abortion itself? What emergency backup is provided—in the clinic itself, or prearranged with a local hospital?

If there is anything else about the clinic that concerns you, ask about that, too. You may have to use a clinic you're not completely happy with. If so, you can supplement the clinic's care with your own resources. You may want to see your own physician before or after the procedure, arrange for a tranquilizer prescription (be sure the clinic is aware of and agrees to this; the staff need to know every medication you are taking at the time of the procedure), arrange to rest near the clinic before going home, and so forth. In the rare event that you have serious concerns about the competence or safety of the clinic, contact the local public health authority and ask whether any complaints have been registered and whether the clinic's license is current. Most of the care described here is required by law.

Getting Away

Do you tell people you are going to have an abortion? Abortion is very common, and completely legal, but some people have strong objections to it. You have to say something to people who are directly affected when you're going to be away from school, work, and family responsibilities. You can tell them exactly what's going on, or just "I have to be away on personal business for a day or two," or give an excuse, such as a trip, a sick relative, or some other medical problem. Remember that untruths do have a way of coming back to haunt you: "What plays did you see on your trip to New York?" "Is your grandmother feeling better now?" "What doctor performed your minor surgery?" You may have been showing signs of distress; people have probably noticed.

If you have children, you also have to consider what to tell them. You have to assume that children 1) suspect something is happening, whether you tell them or not; 2) feel it's shameful if it's secret; and 3) probably can't keep a secret. You will have to have some explanation: "I have to have some treatment from the doctor. I am not sick, though, and I will be fine, but I will need a little rest. Can you help me tomorrow by doing the dishes/reading quietly by my bed/bringing me my slippers?"

Try to arrange to cut back for a few days after your abortion. The vast majority of abortions require only a day or so of recovery. But you cannot know ahead of time how you will feel, physically or emotionally. You can always return to your duties! You can repay your helpers when they need your assistance some time, or even by passing along generosity when some other person needs your help.

What to Bring

Ask the clinic whether you need to bring money with you and whether they accept personal checks, cashier's checks, or credit cards. If the abortion will be covered by your health insurance, bring your insurance card and the required forms for the clinic staff to fill out. Ask whether you have to pay at the time of the procedure and then request reimbursement from the insurance company, or whether the clinic will bill the company directly. You will also want to bring money in case you are given prescriptions for medication and in case you need transportation.

Don't forget to bring the telephone numbers of anyone you may need to call. Some people don't want to try to concentrate on anything before they have a medical procedure. They prefer to sit quietly alone or with someone. Other people get very restless if they don't have something to read or to do with their hands. If you fall into that category, be sure you have a book, magazine, or handwork to do.

Who Can Come With You?

Generally, it is not possible for a friend or relative to be with you during the abortion. The procedure itself is very short, and the treatment rooms are usually just big enough for you and the staff. You can bring someone to wait with you and take you home. There is no rule about who it should be; you can decide. It's helpful to have another person hear the staff's explanations and instructions, but it's perfectly possible, and all right, to go alone if you prefer.

If you have a relationship with the man with whom you created the pregnancy, he is an obvious candidate. Under the best of circumstances, those who began a pregnancy together will see it to its end together, whether the relationship is going to continue or not. On the other hand, you may be pregnant as a result of rape or incest. Regardless of the circumstances, you have no obligation to involve this man if you don't want to. If you are a very young woman, you may want to come with your parents. If they are cold, unavailable, or abusive, you may have decided that it would be best if they did not know about your pregnancy.

Aside from natural relationships between a pregnant woman and the man with whom she created the pregnancy, and between a young woman and her parents, there may be a person who comes to mind when you think of a companion at the abortion clinic. This person may have been supportive and helpful throughout your decision-making process or at other demanding times in your life. What you most likely want and need at this time is a person who is cool-headed, caring, and tolerant. Different women have different preferences. Some women like a chatty, bubbly companion, and others want someone quiet.

Cool-headed does not mean cold. You don't need someone who is more upset than you are. But it's helpful to have someone who is able to express some feelings. The person needs to give you a little tender loving care. You can judge what kind of care, in the range between smothering and ignoring, is most comfortable for you. Some people offer to help but end up demanding attention and care from the people they are supposed to be helping.

Your companion should be tolerant of your needs and feelings. You may experience moments of grief, relief, anger, anxiety, and other emotions. You should not feel you are being stifled or judged.

In Closing

Here is a summary of the suggestions offered in this chapter:

- Anticipate problems (e.g.,anti-choice demonstrators).
- Ask questions.
- Ask again if you didn't get the information you needed.
- Ask for what you need.
- Acknowledge your feelings.
- Give yourself permission to create the circumstances you need.
- Plan to take care of yourself. What would you like to eat, drink, and do after you leave the clinic?

CHAPTER 9

After an Abortion

Your physical condition immediately after an abortion will depend mostly on the stage of your pregnancy and the type of anesthesia used for the procedure. Your general health also plays a role. You will probably feel a bit sore and crampy and may experience some bleeding. The staff will monitor you for an hour or two. In general, you will feel fine.

Emotionally, you will probably be relieved that the whole process—pregnancy, decision, and abortion—is over. You may be in a great rush to leave the clinic and get on with the rest of your life. Give yourself a few minutes to gather your thoughts and feelings. You have just been through a significant life experience. You have found yourself in a difficult situation, you have made an important decision, you have made the arrangements, and you have carried it out.

It is not necessary to push the whole process out of your mind. It is a part of your life, and if you suppress it, your own, internal life story will have a gap. Let your feelings wash over you. They are all okay, even second thoughts and regrets about any step in the process. Everything you have learned is an asset for the rest of your life.

In the unfortunate event that you will have to face anti-choice dem-onstrators as you exit the clinic, prepare yourself. Remind yourself that you have made a choice that women in every walk of life, in every century, and on every continent have made and continue to make, a choice that is accepted by most of the population and by most relig-ious groups. You have undergone a legal, medical procedure. Take a deep breath and go on to wherever you will feel most comfortable and cared for.

You may have planned what you want to do after the abortion is over. Even so, you might be in a different mood than you anticipated. You may have to return to home far away or to get on with responsi-bilities, like schoolwork that will suffer if you miss too much, or child care that others have been covering for you. In those cases, you have little or no choice about what to do after you leave the clinic. Remem-ber to keep a little space in your heart and mind to acknowledge the day's experiences and work with them, little by little, as time goes by. If you are fortunate enough to have some more time at your disposal, try to go with your gut feelings about what you would like to do. There aren't any rules. You might enjoy anything from a movie to cuddling up in bed.

As Time Goes By

Physical Adaptation

Your body will soon heal. You will probably have some cramping and bleeding, more or less like a normal menstrual period. You body will also be adjusting to the hormonal changes from the pregnant to the nonpregnant state. These hormonal changes, like those after the deliv-ery of a baby, can make you susceptible to emotional fluctuations, in-cluding moments of both sadness and happiness.

Physical Signs to Watch For

The clinic staff should inform you what physical signs to watch for. Let the clinic, or your own regular health care provider, know if you run a temperature over 100°F, if you bleed excessively from the vagina (cannot keep up with the flow with your usual menstrual products), or experience significant pain or tenderness.

How much pain or soreness should you worry about? People's sensitivity to pain varies. You know yourself. If you are a worrier, you might wait a little longer before deciding that something is wrong. Abortion is a very safe procedure compared with childbirth and with other surgeries, but call the clinic or your doctor if you are not certain whether your symptoms are something to be concerned about.

If you have prior medical problems, your regular health care provider and the abortion clinic should make some recommendations about recuperating from the abortion. In general, you can do whatever you feel up to doing. It is okay to have enough energy to go out for a walk but not enough to do the laundry. You have been through an emotionally stressful time. Try to find a little peace if you need it. On the other hand, if you cope best when physically active, you should be able to engage in all your regular activities in a few days.

Your Checkup

Having a checkup after an abortion can bring back all the emotions of the abortion just when you are beginning to feel you have put the experience comfortably in the past. Don't allow yourself to avoid or forget your appointment on that account. Having the checkup will officially end the medical aspects of your abortion, reassure you that you have fully recovered, and give you an opportunity to ask questions and get advice about resuming sexual and general activities. The checkup is an essential part of taking care of yourself.

Sex

You may feel certain that you'll never have sex, much less have a problem pregnancy, again. Don't count on it! You can be fertile again within days. Make sure you have contraceptive information and whatever pills or equipment you need. Immediately after the abortion, your cervix (the opening of the uterus) will be more open than usual, and the inside of the uterus will have a healing place that is susceptible to infection. Whatever contraceptive method you use if you have sexual intercourse, you should make sure your male partner uses a condom to protect those areas from infection. This is a time to be particularly careful about putting anything into your vagina.

You don't need to have intercourse to enjoy sex. You can be intimate and can give and receive sexual pleasure by masturbation and many others kinds of contacts and caresses. If feeling close is especially important to you, find a creative, safe, and pleasurable way to do it until you have your checkup.

Your Emotions

Abortion does not cause emotional problems or mental illness.[1] Women do have many feelings before, during, and after abortions. A feeling is not a mental illness. A pregnancy is an important event. After an abortion, a woman is recovering not only from the medical procedure, but also from the difficult circumstances that caused the pregnancy and the need to end it. Youth, financial hardship, emotional abandonment, the breakup of a relationship, responsibilities for other dependents, abuse and violence, and all the other reasons why a problem pregnancy may be begun and ended cause their own emotional stresses.

You will probably handle this situation the same way you have handled similar situations in the past: emotional or businesslike, or some of each. Remember that you always go on functioning after all.

The Reactions of Others

You may have a passing feeling of loss that surprises you. An abortion is a loss regardless of the circumstances. Be prepared for the fact that people who are important to you may not recognize or feel comfortable with any sense of loss. If they have helped you make and carry out your decision, they may not want to accept your ambivalence or sadness. They have invested their caring and their time, and they want to see that your decision made you happy, or at least relieved.

On the other hand, some people may be upset if you are cheerful afterward. Other people's feelings will affect your mood. Some people may behave as if nothing has happened. This can be helpful to you; it gives you the opportunity to concentrate on other aspects of your life, at work or school, for example. At other times, it may make you feel alone. People may bring up the abortion when it is not on your mind. This can help you recognize your own feelings, or it can intrude into your work, your fun, and your relationships.

Other people may not be aware of, or admit to, their own reactions to your abortion. They may be angry, gloating, or curious. You can usually trust your gut reactions and then decide whether to ignore a particular person, stay away from her or him as much as possible, or try to work it out between you. You can explain how the person's behavior makes you feel and how he or she could be more helpful. It's important to let a person who is trying to help know that you appreciate the effort.

You may have feelings of guilt. You may feel you have ended a life, or a potential life. You may feel bad because you did what you thought was best for you. Abortions, and even decisions not to get pregnant, are sometimes called selfish. That doesn't make sense. You have an obligation to take care of yourself and of anyone you're responsible for. Your partner or your parents may feel you've deprived them of a child or grandchild. You don't owe anyone this child, or any child. Remember that a child needs to be wanted by its mother. It is not a gift from its mother to someone else.

Regrets

What about second thoughts, regrets? It is natural to have second thoughts about any major decision. Reflection is a basic, positive human activity. Absolute certainty is not a sign of emotional health. Don't blame yourself for doubting yourself.

Your emotional health after an abortion will probably be about same as it was before. Having an abortion may make you feel normal again, freed of an unwelcome condition. You may again be a teenager, or the mother of adolescent or grown children, fitting in with the mainstream of women your age. Your feelings after an abortion are related to the reasons for your decision to have it. If the conception occurred under particularly painful circumstances, such as incest, rape, or deception, those painful circumstances affect all your reactions. On the other hand, you may be all the more relieved to have the pregnancy behind you.

If you would have liked to continue the pregnancy if circumstances were different, you will be more vulnerable to a sense of loss. If you terminated your pregnancy because of a medical illness or genetic condition, you have to continue to live with them. The abortion reminds you of painful limitations. You might want to join a group of people who have the same problem.

If abortion is against your own religion, you may feel alienated from your faith, your fellow practitioners, and your religious leaders. There are rare instances in which having had an abortion causes a woman to be permanently ostracized from a religious institution. You know best whether you fall into this rare category. If your religious affiliation is a problem, you may want to seek counseling from either a non-affiliated mental health professional or a pastoral counselor of your own or another faith. Generally, even religious groups that forbid abortion will support a woman who felt she needed to choose one. Be alert, though, for groups that make you feel more guilty and that blame all the problems in your life on your abortion. This approach will not help you get on with a virtuous and productive life. These groups have other, political agendas. Look for comfort somewhere else.

Moving On

A wide variety of feelings are normal after an abortion (and after having a baby). Feelings can change from moment, day to day, and year to year. Your life circumstances will develop in both predictable and unpredictable ways that influence your feelings about abortion in retrospect. If this abortion works into your expectations and plans as you had hoped, you will be more satisfied than if your expectations are disappointed. There is no way to know or control everything now. Like everyone else on earth, you can only do your best from day to day.

After the abortion, you no longer face a decision about a pregnancy. You can come to terms with your decision, integrate the decision into your personal life story, and build on your determination to take some control over the direction of your life.

Anniversaries.   The memories and feelings of the abortion may come back on anniversaries of the date of conception, if you know it; the date the pregnancy was diagnosed; the date you would have delivered; and the date of the abortion. These so-called "anniversary reactions" are not specific to abortion; they can happen after any significant life event. The reactions vary from a passing memory or thought to an episode of sadness or anxiety. You may or may not be aware of the link between past events and your experience on the anniversary. The strength of the reaction is related to the reasons you chose the abortion, your feelings at the time of the original events, and the ways in which your life has unfolded since.

The history of your abortion.   As your life goes on, you may be close to different people than the ones in your life now. These people didn't share the experiences of this time, and you may not have told them. Reconsider that decision now and again. Times change. You have new perspectives on the experiences around the time of the abortion. People mature. Of course, you may not trust people you don't know well, who may hurt you. People you know and love will understand and support you better, as you understand and support them, when each of you knows about the important events in each other's past. But be careful.

Health care providers and counselors are sometimes reluctant to ask a woman the details of her reproductive history, including abortion. Whether you are asked or not, you will have to decide whether to tell them about your abortion. You want them to know everything possible about your medical history, and abortion is legal, but they may disapprove. You will have to judge for yourself.

Emotional Risks

Two situations make a woman more vulnerable to an intense emotional reaction or episode of mental illness after an abortion: 1) especially complicated circumstances, and 2) having a mental illness before the abortion. Illegal abortions associated with danger, secrecy, and/or physical pain and complications; pregnancies that occurred as a result of mental or physical coercion; abortions you were pressured into; and traumatic experiences with anti-choice activists as you were making your decision or having your abortion can make an abortion more difficult to deal with emotionally.

If you have had psychiatric illness in the past, there is a small chance that it will flare up now. That doesn't mean that the abortion was the wrong decision or that the abortion itself causes an episode of illness. In most cases, it is the stress of the problem pregnancy itself that contributes to the illness, regardless of whether the pregnancy ends in a birth or in abortion.[2] In fact, in cases of unintended pregnancy, women who choose to continue the pregnancy and give birth to a child may be at an increased risk of experiencing clinical depression.[3]

A mental, or psychiatric, illness is not a mood or a painful feeling that goes away by itself, or with some support from friends and family, in a few hours or days and doesn't keep you from doing things you need and want to do. An illness interferes with your ability to function or requires professional diagnosis and treatment. There are many kinds of psychiatric illness. They include:

- Anxiety disorders—Anxiety or worry for no good reason, or out of proportion to reality; or attacks of terror or panic
- Mood disorders—Prolonged deeply depressed or highly elevated mood, with changes in appetite; sleep; interest in people, in sex, and in other activities; concentration; and energy
- Psychotic disorders—Disturbances in one's sense of reality, such as hearing voices others do not hear or seeing things others do not see
- Somatizing disorders—Preoccupation with physical symptoms or a sense of physical unwellness, even though medical professionals tell you that you are fine.

You may have had a psychiatric illness without recognizing it or without seeking professional care. You may fear that you are losing your mind when you are nervous or stressed. There is a lot of unnecessary misunderstanding, shame, and fear about mental illnesses. Like other medical illnesses, they are caused by a combination of psychological, social, and physical factors.

Probably the most common psychiatric problem after—not necessarily caused by—an abortion is depression. Depression is an extremely common disease; as many as one-third of all people have depression at some time during their lives.[4] Two to three times as many women as men have depression, and young women of childbearing age are particularly susceptible.[5] (Young mothers staying at home with several preschool children have the highest risk of all.) Unfortunately, 80% of people with depression do not get treatment, because they, their loved ones, and their health care providers do not recognize their illness.[6]

Clinical depression is not just a bad mood, and it can't be cured by a change of scene or a new outfit. Depression is linked to changes in the chemical substances that carry messages in the brain. It can be very effectively treated with a combination of psychotherapy and medication that returns the brain chemistry to normal.

Here are the symptoms of depression. Five or more of these symptoms must be present for a significant part of the day, every day, for 2 weeks or more, to constitute clinical depression:

1. Sad mood, often with tearfulness
2. Preoccupation with pessimistic thoughts, including thoughts of death or suicide
3. Decreased energy
4. Decreased ability to concentrate
5. Decreased interest in activities
6. Withdrawal from contact with people
7. Irritability
8. Decreased appetite and food intake, often with weight loss
9. Difficulty staying asleep at night
10. Decreased interest in sex
11. Feeling and acting slowed down or speeded up (agitated)
12. Feelings of self-blame, guilt, or worthlessness

Another kind of clinical depression, which is more common in young people, causes the depressed person to eat and sleep more rather than less than normal.

Depression makes you feel that it's not worthwhile trying to get help and that you're not worthwhile, anyway. It saps your energy. You may have to push yourself to get treatment or may need a push from people who care about you. Treatment works!

Seeking Professional Help

When? If you have previously been diagnosed with a psychosis, a clinical depression, or panic disorder, you should seek help immediately if you think your symptoms are returning or getting worse. Delaying care will not build character; it will make your situation worse and your condition more difficult to treat. If you have never been diagnosed with a mental problem but are suffering emotionally and having difficulty functioning, it is time to seek care.

What kind of care provider do you want and need? There are several basic categories of mental health experts:

- Counselors have training at the college or master's degree level and licensure in some states. They help people with interpersonal problems, decisions, and adjustments to life changes and stress. Pastoral counselors are religious leaders with special training in counseling. Other religious leaders offer counseling to their parishioners as well.
- Most social workers complete a 2-year M.S.W. (Master of Social Work) degree program after college. There are also bachelor's degree programs in social work, and some public agencies designate employees with social responsibilities as social workers without requiring special training. Social workers may specialize in psychotherapy, social policy, or other areas. Many are also knowledgeable about community, state, and federal social programs that may help you to obtain housing, food stamps, child care, or protection from domestic violence.
- Psychologists may be educated at the master's or doctoral (Ph.D. or Psych.D.) degree level. They are experts in the psychological aspects of the diagnosis and treatment of mental illness.
- Psychiatrists are medical doctors whose specialty is mental illness.

They are trained in all aspects of diagnosis and treatment. Because of their medical training, they are the mental health professionals who can prescribe psychiatric medications when necessary and who can treat patients in the hospital.

• Psychiatric nurses are nurses with additional training in psychiatric diagnosis and treatment.

How do you choose which type of professional to consult? You may have a strong preference for or a relationship with a particular provider. More and more often, mental health professionals from different disciplines work together. A psychiatrist, for example, may ask a psychologist to perform psychological tests or a social worker to identify community resources. A psychologist or social worker may consult with a psychiatrist about the need for medication. It is more important to get care when you need it than to worry about which kind of provider to choose.

Finding the care you need. If you do not have a relationship with a mental health professional, you will need suggestions or a referral. You can ask your family doctor or nurse practitioner, your religious leader, or friends or relatives. You can call the nearest major hospital or medical school and ask for the psychiatric service. The psychiatry department generally has practitioners from a variety of disciplines and can arrange for you to have a diagnostic appointment there or refer you to a practitioner in the community. If you are unable to care for yourself or feel that you or anyone else is in danger, go immediately to a hospital emergency department. For non-emergency care, you can also call the state or local professional society of the discipline you have chosen. If you need help with what you think is a serious mental illness, you can also contact the local Alliance for the Mentally Ill or Mental Health Association. They will help your family as well. See the Resource Directory at the end of this book for addresses and telephone numbers of additional mental health resources.

If you are a member of a health maintenance organization or another health care plan, you may be required to consult with a designated primary care provider ("family doctor"), who decides whether you need more specialized help and where you can get it. Don't hesitate to insist on a referral if you need one; appeal the decision if necessary. There are also community mental health centers that provide care on an ability-to-pay basis.

In Closing

Abortion does not cause mental illness, but a stressful situation around a pregnancy can make an existing mental illness worse or, rarely, trigger a new one. Finding mental health care can be difficult. It can require persistence just when you feel as though your energy is depleted. But it's worth it.

SECTION 2

And the People Who Care About Them

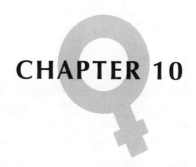

CHAPTER 10

Men and Abortion

There is a man involved in every problem pregnancy and every abortion. The relationship between a man and the woman who is pregnant may be only a single encounter—a one-night stand—or a committed relationship. Even if the man is out of the picture long before the pregnancy is diagnosed, he is important in the woman's decision about her pregnancy. She thinks about having a child fathered by this man, or having an abortion while he suffers no consequences. Some men have difficulty forming intimate relationships; some have sex to prove their manhood or fertility or to try to keep a woman in a troubled relationship.

But many men do care about the pregnancy. They realize that they caused a powerful process inside another human being. The process is mysterious; there is a future child, but nothing to see or feel right now. They feel strongly about their genetic heritage, and they care about their fatherly responsibilities. This chapter is addressed to men who have participated in beginning a pregnancy and who may be facing difficult decisions.

Legal and Moral Perspectives

What are the rights and duties of a man who participates in starting a problem pregnancy? Does he have a right to participate in the decision about an abortion? A man who has caused a pregnancy by rape has no right to participate, but a man who caused a pregnancy in good faith should have the opportunity to discuss, persuade, offer help, and suggest alternatives. Because the pregnancy occurs in the woman's body, however, he cannot dictate the decision. U.S. law upholds this principle.

Two kinds of attempts have been made to establish men's legal rights over abortion. The first approach has been through the courts. Several men, in Canada and the United States, have sued in court to prevent the women they impregnated from having abortions. Although in one case there was an attempt to prevent or delay the abortion during the court proceedings, the attempt failed; the courts have not allowed men to interfere with women's legal rights to abortion. The second approach has been through the passage of laws. The state legislature of Pennsylvania passed a law requiring any married woman to obtain her husband's consent before undergoing an abortion. This law was overturned by the U.S. Supreme Court. Therefore, a man has no legal right to determine the fate of a pregnancy.

According to our laws and our morals, if a woman has a baby, the baby's father must contribute to its support. Some states have laws requiring the mother to name the father, whether she wants to or not, so that the government can require him to provide financial support if their child becomes dependent on public aid. A man may have been purposely misled by a sexual partner who said she couldn't get pregnant. He may have used a condom. Even so, he must support his child. This is a long legal and moral tradition that applies to both parents because of society's mandate that parents care for their children.

Your Feelings

Most men have strong feelings about the termination of a pregnancy that they have had an equal role in conceiving. The pregnancy proves your manliness and fertility and carries on your genes and your family. Deep inside a woman, where no one can see or reach, is a microscopic bundle of cells that may or may not become your child. You may feel guilty about implanting this problem in a woman's body, especially if you seduced the woman into sex with promises of contraception or commitment. On the other hand, you may feel angry and betrayed to learn that a woman is pregnant by you, especially if a woman assured you that you didn't have to worry about contraception. The pregnancy may make you feel helpless and trapped. The decision about the pregnancy will be up to the woman.

Becoming a Father

If you don't want to have this child, but the woman does, you will become a father against your will, with all the legal, moral, and emotional responsibilities of parenthood for the rest of your life. You may attempt to shirk those responsibilities, but they will not go away. The child will tie you legally, biologically, and emotionally to the woman who is now pregnant. This pregnancy, and the birth of a child, can be used to pressure you into leaving another relationship, even another family, or to remain in an unhappy relationship. It can humiliate you in your family, workplace, church, or community.

If you deny that you are the father, you can be forced to have genetic testing. If you are proved to be the biological father, and the baby is not given up for adoption, you will have to contribute financial support voluntarily, be forced to do so by the law, or try to run away. You will have to negotiate with your baby's mother over financial support, visitation, and all your other parental responsibilities. Your plans for your education, career, and family may be affected. All this will be the result of one act of unprotected sexual intercourse or one contraceptive failure. It can be an infuriating, frustrating, and depressing reality.

The two partners in a committed relationship can also have differing wishes about how to deal with a pregnancy. You may feel overburdened by children already born, the needs of other family members, or financial obligations. You may feel that the birth of another child will prevent you from being the kind of parent, son, or worker you should

be. It may destroy your dreams of education, travel, romance, and freedom. On top of everything, you may be expected to be happy about the
coming baby and supportive of your wife or partner. It's difficult to tell
friends and relatives that you wish your child wouldn't be born—and
your child might find out later.

Reactions to Abortion

You may be very relieved if the woman decides to have an abortion. But
you may want the child and be forced to stand by while the woman has
an abortion. You may have strong religious beliefs about abortion. This
pregnancy may be a long-awaited opportunity to start a family. Your
parents may be eager for a grandchild. You may be grieving not only the
loss of your potential child, but the loss of your relationship. The abortion feels like a rejection of you: your genes, your body, your compan-
ionship, your ability to be a father. The woman may be contemptuous,
disillusioned, or angry. You may feel that she will be having an abortion
out of spite.

Because it is a woman who becomes pregnant and has an abortion,
you may feel you have no right to have painful feelings or to get help
with them. You can be supportive of the woman having an abortion
without denying your own feelings. You will be more helpful to her if
you can be honest with yourself.

Coping and Getting Help

Men are generally more reluctant than women to think and talk about
painful feelings. Men are often more likely to throw themselves into their
work, try to drown their sorrows in alcohol, or keep a stiff upper lip.
Think about the ways you usually cope in hard times. What helped before
will probably help again. But some reactions are counterproductive.
Hangovers and drunken driving add to trouble. Running away probably
won't work and might cause years of painful repercussions. A problem
pregnancy can require new coping mechanisms. People often experience
multiple, changing, and conflicting feelings at a time of crisis.

Make sure you have accurate information. Don't rely on someone else's experience or things you might have heard years ago. For example, you may believe that your religion considers abortion a sin, when in fact many religious bodies support reproductive choice. You may think that abortion costs more than you can afford, is illegal, or causes medical complications. You may not be aware of programs to help you if you become a father. Good sources of facts include Planned Parenthood and the American College of Obstetricians and Gynecologists. Resources are listed at the end of this book.

How are your feelings affecting your state of mind and your ability to perform your responsibilities? It is normal to have brief disturbances of sleep, appetite, and concentration during a major life event. People often experience nervousness, preoccupation, and disinterest in friends and pleasurable activities. After the initial shock, or after an event, such as an abortion, has taken place, these disturbances should begin to resolve. If they don't, if the emotional pain is too great, if you have trouble with important relationships or work, or if you just can't make up your mind what to do, it is time to get help.

Friends and Family

Most people look first to friends and family for help in a crisis. But pregnancy and abortion are emotional subjects. You have to think carefully about how people will react, both now and in the years to come. You or the woman involved may want to keep the pregnancy and the decision a secret or to share it with only a very few friends or relatives. You know who's been helpful in the past. On the other hand, most families have faced similar situations. Friends and relatives may be more accepting and helpful than you expect.

Clergy

Members of the clergy provide counseling for difficult life situations and complicated decisions. They can be especially helpful when there is a question of religious laws and practice and if the religious leader is already a trusted and familiar adviser. A religious counselor, in addition to helping you with your feelings and your decision, can help with atonement and forgiveness.

Professional Help

If your main problem is in your relationship with the pregnant woman or some other relationship, joint counseling can be very helpful. Men and women often deal differently with difficult life situations. Sometimes they misunderstand each other. You may keep your feelings to yourself to spare your partner, but she may think you don't care. She may find it comforting to cry on your shoulder, but you may feel worse if she cries every time she sees you. Joint counseling can help you appreciate and understand each other's feelings.

If you are too anxious or depressed to function, you need help for yourself. You can probably benefit from psychotherapy and/or medication. Your family physician can make an assessment, begin treatment, or make a referral to a psychiatrist.

Giving Help

Facing Responsibility

Because it's the woman who makes the decision and has the abortion or the baby, you may feel you have no real part to play. The woman may even blame you for the problem pregnancy and keep you out of the process. It will be good for you to find some way to feel active rather than passive. As an equal contributor to the situation, you have a responsibility to try to help. Your behavior in this difficult time reflects your character and becomes a part of your life history.

Letting Her Know

If the pregnant woman is keeping you away, maybe there is another way to approach her. Ask mutual friends or her friends or relatives how you can help. Send a message or a note through them, letting her know you're concerned and available. Don't give up too easily, but don't badger her, either. You don't have to agree with the decision or make a permanent commitment to the relationship. Dishonesty will cause more problems in the long run.

How to Help

What kinds of help can you provide? You can offer information, company, understanding, transportation, mediation, money. You can make telephone calls to locate a clinic, a doctor, a member of the clergy, or someone who is familiar with local laws and regulations.

Don't underestimate the value of just being there. You can't give birth to a baby or have an abortion, but you can be there, not only for the procedure, but also for the decision making and the recovery. Tell the woman clearly and honestly that you are available—to talk, to listen, to get information, to drive, to hug, to come along. Let her know that you can accept whatever emotions she is experiencing.

Supporting her decision.   You need to let the woman facing this decision know that you will support her decision, whatever it is. This takes a lot of strength of character and emotional generosity. At the same time, you shouldn't deny your own feelings and values. Support means accepting the fact that the pregnancy exists in the woman's body and respecting her right, even her need, to do what she thinks best.

Money.   Money talks. Even when health insurance will pay for an abortion, the offer of financial assistance demonstrates your involvement and responsibility. There are many expenses associated with a problem pregnancy: pregnancy tests, medical examinations, transportation, child care, and loss of income from work, to name just a few. You may feel that, because she has to have all the procedures, you should bear all of the expense. Some women prefer to share the cost, and others want to maintain control by paying for everything themselves. Money can't substitute for other forms of responsibility, though. Whether the money is for an abortion or a child, the woman must not feel that you are trying to "buy her off."

Coming to the clinic.   Try to be at the abortion clinic, hospital, or doctor's office for the abortion. It may feel awkward to sit in a waiting room surrounded by women patients. It seems like an announcement of your role in the pregnancy to a group of strangers. Many people find medical settings very anxiety-provoking. The prospect of a woman to whom you've been close undergoing a medical procedure, and an intimate one, is not an easy one.

Maybe you're worried that she will be sad or angry at you. Maybe you won't know what to say or do. Remember that she, too, is using her coping skills just to get through this process. Encourage her to tell you how she feels and what she needs.

After an Abortion

What you'll probably feel after an abortion is relief. You have weathered a crisis, made a decision, and carried out the decision, and you are ready to get on with your lives. You may have passing feelings of sadness and guilt. Even when a pregnancy is not planned or wanted, or when it's not the right time or place for the birth of a child, the termination of a pregnancy is a loss.

Immediately after the abortion, the woman will spend an hour or more in the clinic, and she will probably be advised to rest for the rest of the day. Be prepared for a wide variety of reactions, from tears to smiles. She may want to stop off for a snack before heading home, or she may want to go straight to bed. She may want to talk or to keep her feelings to herself. She may be grateful or angry. She may want to be alone, with you, or with someone else. All these feelings are normal, and they may change over time.

Outcomes

Men who share in the feelings, decisions, and events connected with a problem pregnancy and an abortion come out of the experience more mature and more in control of their lives than they were before. The problem pregnancy forces you to think seriously about your own behavior and its consequences and to participate in a decision that will have a tremendous impact on your life.

Taking Sexual Responsibility

A problem pregnancy is an opportunity to reassess your attitudes about sex and contraception. It makes you realize the direct connection between making love and starting a pregnancy and the impact of a pregnancy on people's lives. Some men believe that because women get pregnant, women should take care of contraception. But if you don't take responsibility, you have no control over whether a pregnancy occurs. If the problem pregnancy was the result of a failed contraceptive method, you're probably skeptical about contraceptive methods. Consider consultation with an expert.

The last two sections concern situations different from the usual ones. The following section concerns boys and very young men and is addressed to families. The final section is addressed to men who are close to the pregnant woman but who did not participate in starting the pregnancy.

When the Man Is a Boy

Sometimes the man involved in a problem pregnancy is very young. It may be difficult for him to grasp all the implications of the situation. He may be preoccupied with fears about the response of his parents or with pride at his ability to make someone pregnant. He may rush into commitments without being able to understand the long-term consequences, or he may retreat and insist that he doesn't care.

He, like any other man, will have to leave the final decision about the pregnancy to the pregnant woman. Her family may gather around her, pointing the finger at him as the culprit, refusing to allow him to speak with her, or demanding that he marry her. They or others may reveal the news of the pregnancy, exposing him to a variety of reactions by his own friends and relatives. Or they may swear him to secrecy, forcing him to bear the emotional burden of the situation alone. He may stand miserably on the sidelines while a major drama of his young life is taking place.

To have caused a pregnancy is a profound thing. A very young man desperately needs help from his parents or other caring adults at this time. They have their own feelings, too. They may be surprised. The young man has put them, as well as himself, in a painful situation. He has jeopardized his future, inflicted a crisis on a woman, and exposed the family to criticism and financial burdens. If they have given him no preparation for sex, or even encouraged him to prove his manhood by becoming sexually active, they may feel ashamed or guilty. They often feel angry and betrayed.

At the same time, the parents need to help a young man with his feelings. If he is not upset, he should be. He must recognize that parenthood is an awesome possibility and that this possibility is being played out in someone else's body. He needs to be able to talk about his guilt, his fear, his sense of helplessness and loss, and his questions in a supportive atmosphere. Counseling should be made available if he does not seem to be coping well or if he requests it.

Parents shouldn't take over and manage the whole situation. Though he may be young now, it will be much better for him, as he matures, to have done what he could to help. He can contribute money of his own, share in discussions about the decision, and offer to support his partner emotionally. His success or failure in accepting his responsibilities will stay with him.

When the Man Involved Is Not the Father

Sometimes a woman feels more comfortable getting help from a male friend who isn't the biological father of the potential child. This is a special role for a man. If you are this male friend, the situation is bound to provoke feelings about the man who made the woman pregnant and men in general. If you are a male friend or boyfriend, as opposed to a relative, other people may think that you are the potential father. You may even be the woman's husband. You have to deal with the circumstances under which the woman became pregnant; was there an assault, an offer of commitment, an affair? If the woman was a willing partner in the conception, you may be angry and jealous while trying to be helpful. If the woman was attacked or tricked, you are angry, possibly extremely so, and skeptical about other men in general.

If you accompany the woman to the abortion clinic, the staff and the other patients will probably assume that you are responsible for the pregnancy. Either way, it can be embarrassing for you and for her. But above all, your presence is especially important to a woman who has been abandoned and hurt by a man who is unable or unwilling to accept his responsibilities.

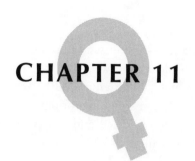

CHAPTER 11

Parents, Other Relatives, and Friends

A problem pregnancy can happen to any woman who can conceive. Because there are some differences between the problems of an adult daughter and those of an adolescent daughter, this chapter has separate sections on each. The term "parents" is intended to refer not only to biological and adoptive parents, but also to other adults who are responsible for a young woman. Special issues for the single parent, as well as for other relatives and friends of the pregnant woman, are also discussed.

For the Parents of a Pregnant Woman

All too often, problem pregnancies occur in teenagers. Parents have to cope with their own feelings while helping their child to think ahead, make a decision, and carry out that decision. There is also a man involved in the pregnancy—a man who may be another youngster, like your daughter, or an older man who has taken advantage of her. You have to use your maturity, experience, and knowledge, not to take over the situation, but to help her weigh her options and make her own decision, because making a supported and independent choice is what is best for her in the long run.

Stages of Adolescent Development

Adolescence covers a wide range of ages and stages. There is a vast difference between an average 12-year-old and an average 19-year-old, and a lot of variation among girls of the same age. Younger adolescents tend to see life problems in black and white. They are still developing the capacity to grasp the long-term implications of their choices and behaviors. They have an exaggerated fear of the reactions of authority figures, especially their parents, to unexpected and unwelcome news.

Some girls are so overwhelmed by the idea of pregnancy that they don't realize they are pregnant. (This can happen to older women as well.) Or they may dread their parents' response so much that they conceal their pregnancies for weeks and months. Parents can also be unwilling to recognize that their youngster could be pregnant. This results in delays, and delays can make the choice of abortion more medically complex, more urgent, or even impossible.

It is difficult for very young people to grasp the 24-hour, day-in-and-day-out responsibilities of parenthood. Even mature adults are surprised by them. A pregnant young woman may have romantic dreams of cuddling a little baby as if it were a doll or stuffed animal. Advanced pregnancy and birth seem unreal and far away. Only after she has a baby does she face the loss of childhood friends, activities, and educational opportunities, along with the realities of caring for a child. Fears of a gynecological examination or an abortion may in the short term overshadow the farther-off realities of childbirth and parenting.

Adolescents may also have romantic notions about love and marriage. They may imagine themselves walking hand in hand on the beach or living in a cozy home with the boyfriend with whom they started the pregnancy. They do not appreciate the financial strains, the limited opportunities for employment, or the difficulty of the young man in giving up his lifestyle for a life as a husband and father. You, too, may look to marriage to the boy or man involved in the pregnancy as a solution to the crisis.

Roles for Parents

Parents are key figures in the lives of very young pregnant women. As a parent, you can help your daughter get information and look realistically at her choices. You can review family values and religious beliefs, along with plans for her education, career, and family. You have a lifelong relationship to draw on. You know her emotions, her relationships, and her styles of coping with stressful situations. She needs information—about medical care, parenting, adoption, abortion. (Sources of information are listed under the "Resources" section at the end of this book.) You can (if you have the money) pay for medical care, travel, and other expenses connected with the pregnancy. You can offer to take care of your daughter and her baby if she chooses to carry the pregnancy.

Parents walk a fine line when helping a child through a crisis. Your daughter needs your help, your resources, and your wisdom. But she also needs the experience of confronting and thinking through her situation, acting on her own behalf, learning to obtain and weigh information, and living with the consequences. A problem pregnancy, as unfortunate as it is, can be a maturational step. Anyone in a crisis can use an advocate, someone who remembers the questions she wanted to ask, the things she wanted to say. Most people find the presence of another caring person deeply soothing at a time of crisis and when undergoing a medical procedure. If your daughter has an abortion, you can ask to be with her for as much of the process as possible.

Parents' Feelings

While doing all of this, you have to cope with your own feelings. This pregnancy may be first indication that your "little girl" was sexually active. If she didn't tell you the truth about it, you feel shocked and betrayed. Even worse is the sense that you must have been out of touch.

You should have known what was going on. Or you may have been aware that your daughter was sexually active. You've warned her to protect herself, but she got pregnant anyway. This may be infuriating.

As the parent of a pregnant teenager, you grieve for the loss of her innocence and youth. She has to make a major, irrevocable life decision and live with the consequences for the rest of her life. She has to undergo medical examinations and procedures. The dreams you've had for her since she was born may now be impossible to achieve. Her own plans may be changed or interrupted. She has to deal emotionally with her relationship with her sexual partner. She may have been seduced, abused, abandoned, or rejected by him. She may be deeply attached to him. It is painful to watch your child suffer.

Your daughter's pregnancy is likely to bring back memories of your own early sexual experiences and romances. Maybe you had a pregnancy in adolescence, one that ended in abortion or the birth of a child. The daughter who is now pregnant may have been the result. You may be deeply sad, or deeply angry, to see your mistake repeated. You may want to spare your daughter whatever suffering you endured, or you may want her to suffer. If you postponed your own sexual activity until after marriage, you may have trouble understanding how your daughter could have gotten into this situation.

Interactions Between Parents

Sometimes a young woman tells one parent about her pregnancy only on the condition that the other parent not be told. It is not easy to decide what to do in this situation. Parents usually know each other's personalities, past behaviors, and beliefs. Still, if you encourage your daughter to share the news with the other parent and there is an unhappy outcome, you will feel guilty and the girl will feel betrayed by the one parent she trusted. If you refuse to respect your daughter's wishes and tell the other parent, with or without telling your daughter, there is the same risk.

You may share the news with the other parent in order to get support and advice but ask the other parent to keep the secret. This puts the other parent in a very awkward position. Lastly, you can respect your daughter's wishes and exclude the other parent from an important event. You will be burdened with a secret, and the other parent may learn the truth one day and feel betrayed, rejected, and furious.

Sometimes news of a pregnancy is shared between parents in anger rather than in a spirit of collaboration: "I told you that girl would get into trouble!" This is understandable, but not helpful. It is all too easy for a daughter to become a weapon for each parent against the other or for her needs to be overlooked as her two parents engage in battle. A young daughter's pregnancy requires that two parents, even after years of estrangement and disagreement, put her first and work together. The final decision about the pregnancy will be up to your daughter. You will all have to live with the outcome for the rest of your lives. If parents are too upset with each other to help their daughter, they should have counseling.

What should parents do when they have an honest disagreement about what their daughter should do? Try very hard to work out a compromise. Parents should be honest about their views and preferences; children can cope with parents' differences from an early age. Bitterness, anger, and competition are another matter. Your daughter mustn't feel that her decision is a matter of loyalty to one parent or the other. Both parents must make it clear that they will love and support her regardless of her decision.

Parents and the Community

Your reactions are also related to your religious beliefs and the standards of your community. Some communities regard an adolescent pregnancy, an abortion, or a teenage mother as a disaster, whereas others accept them as a natural part of life. You may want to consult with your religious leader, both for information and for support. Find a religious leader who will help, not make you feel worse. Chapter 6 has more information about the religious aspects of abortion.

Do you want to try to keep this whole event secret? You probably know your community and how they are likely to respond if they know your daughter is pregnant and is considering an abortion. Secrets are very hard to keep. It is emotionally and practically useful to share your problems, but every person who knows decreases the possibility of secrecy. You can consult a community social worker or community agency like Planned Parenthood to find out what resources are available to help you and your daughter.

There is a delicate balance here. Parents need their own support system. In one sense, you have the right to either share your feelings or keep them to yourself. At the same time, the person who is actually pregnant is your daughter. She may have the same, or very different, feelings about who should know and who should participate. Daughter and parents need to discuss, as early as possible, their feelings about telling other people so as to reach some agreement. Once the news is out, it cannot be retrieved.

Other Children

You may also have other children to think of. There is no way to conceal the fact that something important is happening in the family. You have to decide whether to tell the truth, how much of it, and in what words. You have to weigh the complications of telling the truth against those of lying or denying that anything has happened. How old are the other children? It is possible to be honest without overwhelming them with more information than they can digest. Acknowledge the fact that the family is concerned about something, so that children don't imagine it's something even worse.

This is not the occasion to teach the other children about the dangers of disobeying their parents, dating, or becoming sexually active. They can be told the simple truth: their sister is pregnant, and either she will have a baby or she will end the pregnancy. If children are told, don't expect them to keep secrets. The sense of a dark family secret will strain all their relationships. If the secret slips out, they will feel guilty and frightened. If it is important to the family that the secret be kept, tell the children that something private has happened, that it is not their fault, and that everybody is going to be okay. Acknowledge that you are upset now because someone has hurt their sister's feelings.

A Time for Review and Planning

You must consider why this pregnancy occurred. Was your daughter uninformed about sex, reproduction, and contraception? Was she embarrassed and afraid to ask for information and advice? Was there a place outside the family where she could have gotten that information and advice? Was she informed but unable to put her knowledge into effect? This is not a time for recriminations, but it is a time to consider whether your daughter needs education or counseling, either now or after the immediate crisis has been resolved. As impossible as it may seem now, she is vulnerable to becoming pregnant again. She has to be protected as soon as this pregnancy is over.

A daughter who has become pregnant as an adolescent would probably benefit from counseling, either on her own or with the rest of the family. Parents are usually too close, too emotional, to provide all the help that their daughters need. Your daughter may have a treatable depressive illness, a learning difficulty, or a problem with her self-esteem. She may have been the victim of abuse or exploitation that she can't acknowledge, even to herself. The problem pregnancy is a symptom of problems that can interfere with her development and blight her future. Various people and organizations can refer you to a counselor: your religious leader; family physician or pediatrician; community family or mental health center; state or local psychological, social work, or psychiatric organization; or the child psychiatry service of a medical school.

Dealing With the Man

You probably have strong feelings about the man who made your daughter pregnant. The nature of those feelings will depend on the man's age and character and on how he treats your daughter. You also have to deal with your daughter's feelings about the relationship. After all, it is her pregnancy.

When the man involved is also very young, he will need the advice and support of his own parents. The two young people and the two sets of parents may want to meet to discuss the situation together. The young people may be deeply infatuated with each other and determined to make a life and raise a child together. Or one may want to continue the relationship and the other may want to end it; one may want the pregnancy aborted and the other may want it continued. There may be all kinds of accusations about the relationship and the conception.

Each set of parents may be furious at the other young person, holding him or her responsible for leading their child astray. Each set of parents should support their own child, but accusing the other young person or family of terrible behavior or terrible character will just make the situation more difficult. If a child is born, the two families will be linked forever and will need to get along for the benefit of their children and grandchild. Both sets of parents can help their children to review their finances, their educational objectives, and their living circumstances. They can help them to talk to each other realistically and calmly about the situation. They can help them find resources for information and support.

If the man is older than the young woman, as is very often the case, he may seek to play a role in the decision and the outcome. You will have to judge whether he exploited your daughter and whether his involvement is in your daughter's best interest. Even if it isn't, you have to consider what your daughter wants. Discuss your observations of his behavior and intentions with your daughter. Forcing a young woman to make a choice between her lover and her family is a dangerous gamble. If your daughter chooses her lover, you leave her in his hands.

Often the man concerned is out of the picture in one way or another. Even so, you have to deal with the fact that he was involved in causing the pregnancy and will be the biological father of the baby if the pregnancy continues to term. If he is not aware of the pregnancy, you and your daughter have to decide whether to find him and inform him. Try to make the best possible decision for the long term. If he is not informed, the man may return at an unexpected time to claim parental rights. There has been at least one tragic custody battle under those circumstances. If you contact him, he may legally terminate his parental rights or sign a formal written agreement to support his child. On the other hand, involving him may be more trouble than it's worth.

Realistic Prospects

Unfortunately, the prospects for a marriage and a family founded in a situation like this are grim.[1] The marriages seldom last. The educational and financial futures of a young woman are worse when she is a married mother than when she is a single mother. Her children are at risk for a life of poverty. There are exceptions, of course. You will consider what you have to offer your daughter in the way of financial, social, and emotional support, as well as her personal assets and what she wants to do.

Whose Decision Is It?

Make your preferences clear, and try to spell out exactly what help you can offer your daughter. If she decides to deliver, can you make a commitment to help with the care of a baby? Be realistic; an adolescent mother and her infant in the family home are a major strain on space, resources, time, and emotional energy—not only for the parents, but for everyone in the household. On the other hand, you and the rest of the family may find yourselves more attached to the baby and more willing to help than you expect.

Your daughter must ultimately arrive at her own decision, and you must ultimately do your best to support her. Don't pressure or force her, no matter how much you disagree. She is the one who will have to live through the decision and live with it. Her opportunity to make an independent, supported decision will be the most important factor in her psychological outcome.

Parental notification and consent laws.   Several states have laws requiring that a woman under legal age inform her parents or obtain their consent before she is allowed to have an abortion. There is a more complete discussion of these laws in Chapter 4. These laws are prejudiced in favor of teenage parenthood in that no consent is required for a young woman to continue the pregnancy, deliver the child, and decide either to raise it herself or to allow someone else to adopt it. She has the legal right to consent to medical procedures related to the pregnancy without consulting her parents, and she has complete parental rights over her child if it is born. If her parents do not allow her to make her own decision about an abortion, either because of their personal beliefs or because they do not consider her mature enough to weigh all the issues, they force her into a situation that requires much more maturity than she may possess and over which they will have little control. As they already know, parenthood is one of the most demanding roles in life.

Most young women who are pregnant choose to tell their parents and discuss their decisions with them. When 1,500 unmarried women under legal age who were having abortions were asked recently about what they had told their parents, 61% said one or both of their parents knew about the abortion, 26% said their fathers knew, 57% said their mothers knew but hadn't told their fathers, and 30% of those who did not tell their parents had experienced family violence or feared that it would occur if they informed their parents about their abortions. Of those who didn't tell their parents, 89% consulted their boyfriends, 52% another adult, and 22% a professional adviser.[2]

When a pregnant girl consults a health care professional, the physician, nurse, or counselor will offer to help her tell her parents and to arrange a meeting with her and her parents if she wishes. But professionals must also respect her confidence if she fears that involving her parents will result in abuse or abandonment.

Judicial bypass. In states that require parental notification and/or consent for abortion for underage women, there must be a provision for "judicial bypass." This means that the young woman can go to court, where a judge will determine whether she is mature enough to make a decision on her own. These provisions are enacted so that young women with abusive or neglectful parents may obtain abortions without provoking physical punishment or exclusion from the family home. Unfortunately, they demand an unreasonable amount of knowledge and sophistication, threaten a young woman's confidentiality, and are unevenly applied from state to state. (See Chapter 4 for a further discussion of judicial bypass.)

Pregnancy resulting from assault or incest. If your daughter's pregnancy is the result of sexual assault or incest, you and your daughter must deal with a crime as well as a pregnancy. Professional counseling is indicated. When the culprit is a stranger, the family must deal with the feeling that they have not somehow protected their daughter from harm. They must also face the police and criminal proceedings. If the man has not been caught, you must deal with the horrible realization that he is at large. If he has been caught and is to be prosecuted, your daughter must identify him and testify in the case. There will probably be many hearings. The pregnancy is also a special burden because of its association with an assault.

If the man who impregnated your daughter is known to, or a member of, the family, you have an even more complicated burden. You have been betrayed by someone you trusted. You must face a reality you may have denied or avoided. Don't blame your daughter for not telling you earlier or for telling the truth now. If your daughter won't reveal the identity of her sexual partner, consider the possibility of abuse or incest. Your daughter's welfare must take precedence over protection of the abuser and the family secret. Fathers, brothers, uncles, and cousins can and do make young women pregnant. Your daughter must have protection and professional care. Without them, there are risks of suicide and other destructive outcomes.

The Single Parent

The situation of the single parent depends somewhat on whether that parent is the mother or the father, and on whether the second parent is alive and available. The single parent, whether mother or father, whose adolescent daughter becomes pregnant must deal with the feeling that fate has presented him or her with yet another parenting crisis to cope with alone. Either parent must deal with the fact that a man has impregnated his or her daughter, but this fact provokes different feelings in each parent. A father is the same sex as the daughter's sexual partner. If you are the father, you may feel ashamed on behalf of your whole sex.

If you are the mother, the crisis of the pregnancy may reawaken the circumstances of your separation from your daughter's father, with bitterness toward men in general. You have to distinguish between your own situation and that of your daughter. Telling a young woman that her lover is "no good like your father" will not help.

The single parent faces a particularly delicate situation with regard to confidentiality. You have no spouse to confide in. You have to weigh the risks of gossip and criticism against the benefits of finding someone to listen and provide support. Many single parents imagine that, if only the other parent were physically or emotionally available, the other parent would know just what to do and say. It isn't a matter of gender; it may be either "a girl needs her mother at a time like this" or "where is a father when you really need him?" On the other hand, a single parent does not have to deal with the feelings and preferences of a second parent. One helpful parent is enough to help a young woman through this episode.

You may feel vulnerable to criticism because the daughter has grown up in a "broken home" or "dysfunctional family" or simply without two parents. But just as this is not a time to blame your daughter, it is not a time to blame yourself. The better you feel, the more you will be able to help your daughter. The pregnancy cannot be undone, but your love and support can have a tremendous impact. If you are too upset to be helpful or the crisis is damaging your own emotional health, get professional counseling.

Problem Pregnancy in an Adult Daughter

There is no magic dividing line between adolescence and adulthood. Some 17- and 18-year-olds are independent and mature; some women in their 20s—and 30s and 40s—are very dependent on their parents. A daughter of any age can benefit from the understanding and support of her parents, but an adult daughter may or may not choose to call on that support, and her parents may or may not be willing or able to give it. After a daughter reaches the legal age of majority, parents, in most instances, no longer have authority over or responsibility for her medical care. The involvement between parents and adult daughters depends on the individuals and the circumstances, without any specific guidelines.

Of course, parents are parents, no matter how old their child is. Events, relationships, and decisions in your daughter's life provoke powerful parental feelings: proud, happy, sad, and mad. Daughters are their parents' children throughout their own adult lives as well. They have intense wishes and feelings about their parents. They look to them as role models and for love and support.

A daughter's problem pregnancy adds another twist to the relationship. There is the possibility of a grandchild. This may be something you've been hoping for, or the last thing on earth you want. You may think your daughter is too poor, immature, or unsettled to be a good mother. If your daughter stays pregnant, you will be a grandparent. If your daughter chooses adoption, you won't know your grandchild or where he or she is. If your daughter raises the child, you will have a strong emotional investment in him, or her.

Here are some points to consider:

- What has your daughter asked from you?
- Are there things your daughter may want but be reluctant to ask for?
- Should she find other resources to help her, rather than involving you?
- Can you help, or are you too angry or exhausted to be constructive?
- Can you respect and support whatever decision she makes?
- Do you want to influence your daughter's decision for reasons of your own?
- How are you going to feel about this situation months and years from now?

Listen at first, without offering opinions or advice. This is one of the most powerful but underestimated forms of help one person can give another. Listening allows the other person to review her own values, wishes, and circumstances. She may realize what she wants to do. Ask her what help she would appreciate and let her know that you will be supportive and available.

Being There, and Other Things to Do

Just being there is comforting to most people going through a life crisis. Your daughter may hesitate to impose on you. Let her know that you would be happy to be with her or go with her to a clinic. Respect her need to be left alone if she wishes. You can also be helpful by getting information, providing transportation, offering financial assistance, baby-sitting, and helping out at home.

When You Find Out Afterward

Sometimes a daughter decides to make a major decision without telling her parents. You may learn about her abortion later, from her or from someone else. You may feel hurt because you were excluded, angry because you would have disagreed with her decision to have an abortion, dismayed because you would have liked to have helped, or relieved that it is all over, or have all of these reactions. The challenge is to respect your daughter's need and right to do what she thought best and go on from there. You can ask why she didn't tell you beforehand. You may not like what you hear, but don't be defensive. You don't have to agree, but respect her feelings and appreciate her perspective. Painful events offer opportunities to improve relationships.

After a Daughter's Abortion

Women who have abortions react in many different ways. The predominant feeling is usually one of relief, but people also experience temporary feelings of guilt, sadness, and anger. Having a strong sense that the abortion was the right thing to do does not mean that the abortion is not a loss. As in so many other circumstances, parents have to be prepared for anything. Your daughter may seem entirely unaffected and eager to get on with her life, or she may be subdued or even angry. A young adolescent especially may be worried about how her parents are going to treat her. Will she still be your little girl?

Even if you are angry and disappointed, everyone will feel better if you can tell your daughter that you will always love her. All daughters care about their parents' opinions, whether they admit it or not. Older adolescents may be preoccupied with their peer groups or boyfriends and the impact of the pregnancy and abortion on their relationships with them. Older daughters may feel that relying on their parents at a difficult time threatens their independence.

The most important thing is to keep the lines of communication open. The key is listening rather than talking. Make your daughter feel safe to express her feelings without fear you'll judge her or jump to conclusions. If she has little to say, tell her you'll be available whenever she wants to talk about what she has just been through. Let her know that abortion is a significant event but not a catastrophe.

A Final Note for Parents

A daughter's problem pregnancy can be a major stress for parents, calling to mind and heart all the events, hopes, and disappointments of their parenting from conception onward. Like other parental crises, it demands extraordinary generosity, sensitivity, maturity, tact, and self-control. It is in your best interest as a parent to help your daughter despite your confused and negative feelings. Of course, parents are not saints, and even saints are strained under difficult circumstances. Crises also demand self-understanding and self-forgiveness.

Other Relatives and Friends

Your Own Reactions

When you learn that a friend or relative is experiencing a problem pregnancy, you have many feelings, from tender concern, to rage at her male partner, to anger at her for allowing the pregnancy to happen, to jealousy at the attention she may be getting. Much of the information in other sections of this book will be useful to you. Male friends and relatives should also see Chapter 10, "Men and Abortion."

This situation may remind you of a problem pregnancy in your own past. You can be helpful even if you are disappointed, jealous, or angry, but not if you are hiding those feelings from yourself. They will show up one way or another. Knowing your own feelings and remembering your experiences will allow you to help your friend or relative more effectively. If you can't be helpful right now, explain that you will stay away until you can.

Deciding How to Help

Does your friend or relative need money, information, help with child care, or transportation to medical appointments or an abortion clinic? Perhaps there is some tension between her and her partner or her other relatives and friends. You may be able to mediate or to explain her feelings and wishes to other people she cares about. Often the most useful things you can do are to listen and be there.

The experience you've already had with your friend or relative will help you know what to do. If she has strong emotions and anxieties, you may be most helpful by staying low key. Remind her that she can think through this situation, make the appropriate decision, see the decision through, and get on with her life. If she is the sort of person who keeps her troubles to herself and hates to bother anyone, be more assertive about offering your help, saying "I'm just going to stay here with you tonight," or "I am going to call my doctor and get some information and advice." Offer to listen, but don't push her to be more openly emotional than she's comfortable being.

What Not to Do

Don't tell your friend what to do. You can help her to get information or to get in touch with people who have been through similar phases in their lives. You can tell her what you would do under the same circumstances. But she will have to live with her decision, and she must make it. Do not tell her what to do even if she asks you. If you do, she may resent it later, blame you for the outcome, or doubt her own competence.

Don't violate your friend's confidence. A problem pregnancy is a weighty piece of news that has the power to change other people's attitudes and behaviors toward your friend now and for years to come. The same is true of an abortion. News travels fast and far; make one lapse and many people will know. That will hurt your friend. Soon your friend will also know who revealed the secret. That will be the end of your friendship.

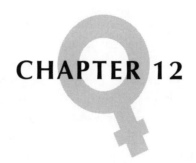

CHAPTER 12

For the Professional Counselor

This chapter is intended for the professional counselor—the religious leader, marriage and family counselor, school or guidance counselor, employee assistance program professional, psychologist, social worker, or psychiatrist—working in an abortion clinic or another setting. Throughout this chapter, I refer to counselors as "she" because most abortion counselors are women. I also refer to all facilities where abortions are performed as "clinics" and to women receiving counseling as "clients."

A counselor may be working with a woman specifically around the problem pregnancy or may have an ongoing therapeutic relationship when the pregnancy occurs. The counselor can provide or help the woman locate necessary information, find and evaluate abortion providers, help the woman think through her decision, and identify psychological conflict and illness when they complicate the process.

Counselors also deal with more complex situations, such as genetic and medical indications for abortion, gatekeeping, and pregnant women with mental disorders. An abortion counselor has to work within a very limited time frame. The counselor has to decide how active a role to take in the decision process. Are there times when she will advise a woman to have an abortion or not to have one, or advise the abortion provider not to perform one? What is the counselor's job, for whom does she work, and what authority does she have? The counselor needs to clarify these issues for herself, and the woman to be counseled deserves to know.

Much of the material in this chapter is covered in the foregoing chapters of this book but from different perspectives. This chapter includes and summarizes those issues that are particularly relevant for counseling.

The Counselor and the Abortion Provider

A counselor may work for a family planning or abortion clinic, at an agency that refers clients for abortion services, or in a general medical or mental health setting. It is enormously helpful for the counselor to be familiar with the other facilities and health care providers that serve her clients. Though she can't assume that clients will react as she does, she can gather information to help clients make choices and prepare them for their abortion experiences. The counselor can establish relationships with clinic staff members to facilitate collaboration in the care of clients. Referring a client by name to a particular person, whether to a receptionist, a nurse, or a physician, lends a warm and personal touch. The counselor can collaborate with the abortion clinic staff around issues raised by particular clients, such as specific fears or difficult relationships, and will have a line of communication for the exchange of information about practices and changes both at her institution and the clinic.

The counselor should attempt to make arrangements for clients to visit clinics before their abortions if they wish to do so. This may not always be possible because of geographic distance or clinical overload at the facility, but it is reassuring and informative. The counselor should also get feedback from women after their abortions: Were the procedures as they expected? Were the staff competent? Supportive? Do they have suggestions for improvements in the services provided by the clinic or the counselor?

Building personal relationships with or working for providers of abortion, adoption, or obstetric services can be a double-edged sword for the counselor. She will become very knowledgeable about the clinic but she will be prejudiced toward it. Is the counselor free to provide unbiased information about the nature and quality of services? Is she free to help women make their own reproductive decisions, or is she expected to convince women to make a particular choice? Are the purposes and biases of the facility made clear to potential clients? Can she be honest about the staff of an office or institution that pays her salary or refers clients to her? Would the clinic staff be upset with her if a woman decided in the course of counseling not to use the services at that institution? Can the staff make constructive use of the counselor's and clients' observations and suggestions about the functioning of the facility?

Counseling based on one particular belief system can be appropriate in a setting devoted to that belief system. For example, a religious group opposed to abortion might offer pregnancy counseling to its members. Such counseling centers should be clearly identified so as not to mislead women who are not familiar with the group. To do otherwise is indoctrination, not counseling. Legal action has been taken against groups that have misled women in this way. The counselor needs to clarify these issues in her thoughts, her feelings, and her practice with clients. If she is a member of a professional society, she can consult with that society about their guidelines for ethical practice. She can also consult her own lawyer.

Self-Evaluation

A counselor has to review her own background, religious and philosophical beliefs, values, and experiences concerning pregnancy, childbirth, parenthood, and abortion in her own mind. The client should be able to expect the counselor to help her arrive at an independent decision. If the counselor has prejudices for or against a particular course of action, those prejudices must be made clear in advance.

Even the most open-minded and professional counselor is a human being with a history, values, and feelings. These qualities are essential for the job, in fact; they can help the counselor empathize with other people's histories, values, and feelings, even when they are different from hers. The relationship between the counselor's and the client's backgrounds and attitudes influences the counseling process in complex ways.

Similarities between the age, race, socioeconomic status, education, ethnicity, and perspectives of counselor and client can help them to understand each other and work together, but they can also lead the counselor to over-identify, to assume the client should or will make the same decision the counselor would have made. Differences between the client and the counselor make them work harder but prevent those kinds of assumptions. Counselors must also be aware of assumptions they might make about the backgrounds, attitudes, and decisions of clients on the basis of race, neighborhood, or other characteristics.

The counselor has to recognize her own attitudes so that they do not unconsciously contaminate the counseling work. This, too, is an enormous challenge because the situations she will confront in her work will repeatedly tempt her to impose her preferences on the decisions of her clients. Actually, such objectivity is not a challenge but an impossibility, a goal toward which she always strives but never reaches.

Certain experiences and values are particularly relevant to the counseling process: the counselor's family's attitudes toward sex, pregnancy, abortion, and parenting as she was growing up, as well as her perception of adult family members' experiences with them. Was her own birth planned? Accepted? Welcome? How did her own mother experience motherhood? Did her mother have fewer or more children than she would have liked? Did she have one or more abortions, either legally or illegally, and under what circumstances? Because abortions were probably not discussed in her family, the counselor may have to piece together the family abortion history on the basis of circumstantial evidence. What kind of a mate and parent was her father?

What are the counselor's own experiences concerning religion, sex, contraception, conception, birth, parenting, and relationships with men? Counselors who have never experienced sexual coercion or contraceptive failure may have difficulty understanding how these not uncommon events could befall their clients. The last thing a woman with a problem pregnancy needs is implied or expressed criticism from her counselor.

We all have strong feelings about parenting. All counselors have been children, and some have children. Each may view parenthood as a blessing, a burden, or some of each. Each may consider a father in a child's home a necessity, a bother, or some of each. Each will have personal criteria for mothers: an appropriate age, marital status, personality, education, living circumstances, income, and social relationships. The client is making a decision about whether to become a parent. There will be times when the counselor hopes a particular client will become a mother and times when she prays that a client will end her pregnancy. The counselor has to keep an inner eye on the impact of her personal feelings and preferences on the counseling process.

Obtaining and Providing Information

Information is never value free. The counselor can offer information to address clients' individual questions. The counselor in an abortion clinic will want to make sure that every client understands what services the clinic provides, how much they cost, what forms of payment are accepted, and what procedures are followed.

Before providing information, it is necessary to get to know the client. Trying to counsel someone about whom the counselor has no information is like talking to someone without knowing what language she speaks. Some of the information the counselor needs to know about the client is:

- How old is she?
- Is this her first pregnancy?
- If she has been pregnant before, what were the outcomes of the other pregnancies?
- What is her marital status?
- What is the status of the relationship in which the pregnancy was begun?
- What are her family and social supports?
- What education has she had?
- What is the nature of her religious beliefs?
- What are her life circumstances, aspirations, and plans?
- How does she feel about becoming a mother—in the past, present, or future?

Why Counseling?

Many of these questions are highly personal, even intimate. What gives the counselor the right to ask them?

There is considerable controversy about the place of counseling in the abortion process. Some argue that counseling should be a required part of the abortion process so that every woman contemplating abortion will have the opportunity to discuss her decision with a trained expert. Others argue that required counseling assumes that women can't make independent, mature, rational decisions about problem pregnancies. It also implies that the decision to have an abortion is potentially catastrophic in a way that other major life decisions are not. Counseling is not required before marriage, before childbirth, or before major, life-threatening medical procedures.

There is a close similarity between abortion counseling and the process underlying informed consent. Before any significant medical treatment, the medical team is required, by law and by medical ethics, to provide sufficient information so that the patient knows the nature of the problem that the treatment is intended to correct, the nature of the proposed treatment and any relevant alternatives, and the risks and benefits of each of these treatments and of doing nothing. Information must be provided in a form that is comprehensible and meaningful to the individual patient. Pre-abortion counseling, at its best, is the optimal fulfillment of the mandate that a patient give informed consent before a medical procedure.

It will be helpful for the client to imagine herself a week, a month, 6 months, a year, 5 years, and 20 years from now, having had an abortion and having had a baby. Where will she be living? What will she be doing? Is she taking steps to reach her life goals? How will this decision affect them?

What does the client want to know? Information that doesn't address the issues about which a person is concerned doesn't register. What are her fears? She may have heard that the clinic's fee is high; while the counselor is explaining other aspects of the process, she may be doing mental arithmetic, dreading the announcement of the price. Clients may be preoccupied with concern about pain during the procedure, fear of anesthesia, or the length of time they will have to miss work or school. They also have concerns about confidentiality. The counselor can state at the beginning of the interview: "What is the question that is most on your mind right now? No question or concern will seem weird or trivial to me."

Many women have been exposed to misinformation about abortion from anti-choice groups, friends, or family members. Common forms of misinformation include gross exaggerations of the medical complications of abortion, including cancer and sterility; and allegations that abortion frequently causes serious psychiatric illness and/or difficulty with mothering, leading to child abuse and neglect. Women may believe that all religious groups are opposed to abortion, that only certain classes of women have abortions, that abortion is illegal, or that abortion constitutes genocide for their race. They may have heard that abortion will cause agonizing pain for themselves and/or the embryo.

The Context of the Client

Cultural considerations. Sensitivity to the individual patient's culture and ethnicity is an important component of counseling. Although the United States contains countless social subgroups and far too many linguistic groups to be specifically targeted and served by any one clinic or counselor, a clinic or counselor can and should obtain information about the predominant groups in the geographic area it serves and provide counseling and printed materials in the languages spoken by those groups, if at all possible.

Pregnancy, childbirth, motherhood, adoption, and abortion have different implications in different cultures. Although each woman experiences her culture in her own way, she does come to counseling with a general cultural background and assumptions.

Religion is often a major component of culture as it relates to reproductive decisions. It is important for the counselor to know something about the religions mostly widely practiced in the area, particularly with respect to religious rules concerning reproduction and abortion, and to identify religious leaders who are open and helpful to clients struggling with religious questions.

Gender role expectations and family structures have powerful effects not only on reproductive decisions, but also on the ways women present themselves for counseling and make use of it. Many Americans are recent immigrants, barely acculturated to mainstream American customs and behaviors. A woman's husband, mother, or mother-in-law may be the determining factor and spokesperson in her reproductive decisions. Having a child under the "wrong" circumstances can threaten her family's social standing and even her life. Having children of one gender or the other may be imperative. Having children may be the only route to social status now and support in old age.

Avoiding unwarranted assumptions. Try to avoid making assumptions. An individual client may come from a certain ethnic group but may not practice the religion of that group. A client may be indigent but very well educated. A client may have a learning disability or mental retardation without any outward manifestation. A client may appear too young or too old to be pregnant. The client may be married but pregnant by a man other than her husband. Or the client may be homosexual or bisexual. Do not assume particular relationships between the patient and the person(s) who accompany her to the clinic. The person who appears to be her "father" may be her sexual partner, or her "sister" may be her lesbian partner.

Identifying assault, incest, and abuse.   It is a particularly impor-tant—and delicate—matter to determine whether the pregnancy has been created in the context of incest, abuse, or violence. Confidentiality is a major issue. The patient's physical or emotional safety may be at stake. Women and children who are abused are frequently ashamed and secretive. They blame themselves for their victimization and are of-ten blamed by their families and society at large. It is useful to have ma-terials about domestic violence openly but discretely available. The materials should be disguised so that they do not provoke the abuser. A client who is not ready to talk about her situation now may make use of the materials and discussion to find help later.

Abusers often threaten renewed violence if the past abuse is re-vealed. An abused woman often lives a constricted life, prevented by a jealous, possessive, or frightened abuser from participating in friend-ships or even from going out of the house. Often the only place she is allowed to go is to the health care setting. The abuser may accompany her and hover closely to monitor what is done and said. This close at-tention can appear to be tender and loving. The abused woman is often depressed and confused and has chronic or repeated stomach aches, pelvic pain, and headaches. She may avoid eye contact, and her stated reasons for wanting an abortion may be unconvincing.

The abused client should be referred for specialized social and psy-chological services. She is at risk of lasting psychological damage, fur-ther injury, and death—risks that she herself may deny. These clients' real-life stories are difficult for friends, relatives, and health profes-sionals to stomach, and they often precipitate denial and rejection.

In some states, the fact that a pregnancy was caused by rape or in-cest is a criterion for funding for or access to abortion. Document the facts carefully in the confidential medical record. The law requires the reporting of abuse or neglect of minor children. Pregnancies in girls under age 15 should arouse suspicion.

Coercion. Even when there is no overt physical or psychological abuse, a client may be seeking an abortion under duress of one kind or another. She may have been threatened with expulsion from her church if members learn that she has become pregnant outside of marriage. Her parents or other friends or relatives with whom she lives may have indicated that she will not be allowed to remain in the household if she brings a new baby into it. If she already has children, her decision could cost them their home as well. Her husband or boyfriend may have stated an intention to leave the relationship if she continues this pregnancy. This, again, could deny existing children a parent and financial support.

Someone may be trying to coerce a client into continuing her pregnancy. Her husband or parents may be opposed to abortion on religious grounds or may feel that it is her responsibility to carry a pregnancy to term. They may even be spiteful for one reason or another. Her male partner may wish to use the pregnancy as a means to keep her dependent and in the relationship against her better judgment or her wishes. Perhaps her family or partner does not even know she is pregnant, and she wishes to have an abortion before they find out.

The client has to weigh the realities of the situation and her own wishes against the preferences and pressures of others. For example, the threat of losing one's housing is a realistic factor for the patient herself, but someone else may be making that threat in order to force the patient either to continue or to terminate her pregnancy. The emotional pressure may exaggerate the danger of the threats in the client's mind, making her feel that there is no alternative but to obey the dictates of the other person or group.

Generally speaking, it will be much better for the patient in the long term if she does what she herself feels is best. The counselor can help her to distinguish her emotional reactions from the specifics of the situation. Housing can usually be found. Relationships based on coercion are seldom in the long-term interests of the woman or her children. Many women who doubted their strengths and abilities have managed to have abortions or to bear and raise children on their own, if that is what they felt was right. The counselor can offer to see or to refer the client for family or marital therapy in an effort to resolve the disagreement.

The Young Client

There is no essential difference between counseling an adolescent and an older woman, except that the counselor and the provider will make an active effort to help the young woman involve her parents or guardian if she has not already done so. Adolescents may imagine that their parents will react more strongly and negatively than they actually will. Most adolescents choose to inform their parents about an abortion, the more so the younger they are. Most parents are helpful. The counselor will offer to help the client to inform her parents and to meet with her and them to discuss her options. The choice should be ultimately that of the young client. She is the one who will become a mother if she does not have an abortion.

Some young women do not wish to, and should not, tell their parents about their pregnancies or abortions. Physical and sexual abuse and neglect of young women are common in all subgroups of society.[1] The young woman who is at risk of abandonment or injury needs help from the counselor to obtain an abortion, if she wishes, without involving her parents.

Providing Information

What the counselor needs to know. The counselor, though not necessarily a medical professional, will need to know in detail the procedure, benefits, and risks of abortion and its alternatives, both in general and in the specific setting in which she works. She will also need to have information about referrals for obstetric and adoption services. The division of responsibility for providing information should be clearly spelled out between the counselor and the staff who actually perform the abortion. The counselor may defer answering some of the client's questions until she can consult the abortion provider or may refer the client directly to the provider for an answer. The counselor should also participate in meetings of the clinic staff in order to offer her perspectives and stay abreast of changes in procedures. The counselor should also confer regularly with the provider to remain current about medical techniques and about the manner in which the provider interacts with patients.

What the client wants to know. Common questions posed by clients considering abortion include the following:

- Are there likely to be people demonstrating outside the clinic, and if so, are escorts available to accompany her?
- How much time will each step of the process take?
- Does the clinic accept personal checks or credit cards, or does it bill clients or insurance companies?
- What forms of identification and what insurance forms should the client bring along?
- Is there an opportunity to meet the provider before the procedure begins?
- Is there a choice of anesthesia? Will she be awake, asleep, or mildly sedated? What should she expect to feel?
- Who will be present during the procedure?
- Can a friend or relative be with her?
- Should she bring a nightgown, sanitary pads, or a book to read?
- When will she be able to resume her regular activities and responsibilities?
- Will she need someone to take her home and to stay with her there?

Clients' interest in and ability to absorb information about a medical procedure vary widely. The inevitable anxiety surrounding a medical procedure can make it more difficult to retain information. That's one reason why it is so important to begin with the client's concerns rather than a standard explanation. Someone who is worried that abortion may make her sterile cannot pay attention to a description of the technical aspects of the procedure. Tell the client explicitly that she will not be expected to remember every detail and that you expect her to need to have information repeated and to have questions.

Most clients worry about taking up the time of overloaded care providers. They are concerned about appearing stupid or unsophisticated. They sometimes indicate that they understand an explanation when they don't. Health care professionals frequently use technical medical language without realizing it. The only way to know that a client has understood something is to have her explain it back to the counselor.

Invite the client to choose a friend or relative to include in the explanation process. The other person is likely to be less anxious than the client, and two heads are better than one. The two of them can discuss the material later to clarify it for each of them. Printed and audiovisual materials are also useful. Some people learn best by listening, others by looking, and still others by reading. Each medium reinforces the others.

Clients' approaches to life events vary, too. Some deal with it by gathering as much information as possible. This will mesh with the counselor's mandate to provide information. But other people prefer to deal with stressful situations by putting them out of mind. They want to make a decision, put themselves in trustworthy hands, and concentrate on other things until it is over. When offered information, they may say: "I'm sure the staff know what they are doing," or "Do we have to talk about that? I'm squeamish," or "I don't want to know all the details." Taken to excess, this attitude can interfere with the client's informed decision making. But for many people, this is not "denial" but a workable way of coping. Ask the client how she usually deals with medical situations. If her behavior now is out of character, or has caused problems in the past, it requires further exploration by the counselor.

Government mandates.   Some states have passed laws requiring that health care providers make specific statements to women considering abortion. The statements include information about the stages of prenatal development, the availability of state funding for prenatal and obstetric care, and the existence of laws requiring biological fathers to provide for their children. The U.S. Supreme Court having upheld some of these laws, counselors are bound to obey them. Nevertheless, they run counter to the intent and process of counseling, which is to exchange desired and useful information in words that are meaningful and understandable to the client. The client has a right to know that the statements are mandated by law and that the counselor will explain and answer questions afterward.

Special information for minors.   In states with laws restricting the access of underage women to abortion services, the counselor will have to know about requirements for parental notification, parental consent, and the judicial bypass process. This information includes which court hears the cases and when, as well as the criteria by which cases are decided. Generally, the client will have to demonstrate that her parents are abusive, neglectful, or unavailable; that she is living independently; and/or that she is mature enough to make the decision for herself. In some states, nearly all requests for judicial bypass are granted, and in others, nearly all are refused. A counselor located in one of the latter states may be able to save a young client a fruitless and demoralizing effort.

Information about quality of care.   The counselor is in an awkward position at times. There may be things about the operation of her own clinic or of other clinics in the area that are not ideal, such as the doctor, the fees, or the techniques. The counselor may not want to endorse any particular clinic because it is not possible to monitor them. The client, for reasons of geography or finances, may have only one choice. The counselor can help the client to prepare for the realities of her care without either making excuses for the provider or frightening her. Any facility that does not meet minimum standards of care should be reported to the state licensing agency or board of health.

Gatekeeping: The Counselor's Role in Access to Abortion

The role of gatekeeper creates a conflict of interest for the counselor. In order to help the client make up her own mind about her course of action, the counselor has to encourage her to reveal and discuss any thoughts, feelings, and circumstances that are relevant to the decision. But if the counselor has the authority to deny access to abortion, the client won't want to say anything that might keep her from getting an abortion if she wants one. The counselor must tell the client at the outset whether the counseling process may result in a denial of abortion services. On one hand, the right to consent to or refuse the procedure is ultimately the patient's. On the other, health care providers are generally not required to perform procedures that they feel are not in the patient's best interest or that contradict their beliefs or professional roles.

Unfortunately, the history of abortion and other reproductive interventions for women is one of authoritarian control rather than informed choice. Having only barely and partially emerged from this history, many women bitterly oppose gatekeeping of any kind. However, some providers argue that they are accountable for their professional work and therefore have the right to evaluate patients' suitability for abortion as for other medical procedures.

There are few, if any, physical contraindications to abortion; a woman who is well enough to bear a child is well enough to undergo an abortion. Concerns about suitability, therefore, are likely to be social or psychological—the very issues the counselor deals with. Counselors need to consider whether to accept this burden. The client who is denied an abortion will go on to deliver a child unless she obtains an abortion elsewhere, legally or illegally.

A client's inability to make a considered decision is a major gatekeeping concern. Such an inability may result from psychosis, extreme anxiety, depression, coercion, or abuse. The counselor should explain her concerns to the client. When the patient and counselor cannot resolve the impasse after working together, the counselor might require that the client give the matter more thought, consult with others (a religious adviser, for example), or obtain additional information and then return in a few days to discuss the decision again. A patient who may have a mental disorder *that prevents her from making an informed decision* (not merely any psychiatric disorder) should be referred to a psychiatrist for evaluation.

Family Planning for the Future

A client's pregnancy may have resulted from unprotected sex or a failure of a contraceptive method. It can be frustrating for counselors to see clients with problem pregnancies day after day. Sometimes it's difficult to understand how so many of these pregnancies could occur. Therefore this part of the work requires special empathy and tact. Making a woman feel stupid or sloppy will not help her with contraception and protection from sexually transmitted diseases in the future.

Inhibitions about using contraception and difficulties refusing sex are common in women of all social classes and levels of education. There are understandable concerns about the side effects and complications of oral contraceptives and intrauterine devices, squeamishness about touching one's own body to insert diaphragms and contraceptive substances, and awkwardness about discussing these matters with one's sexual partner. Many women have limited access to gynecological services, responsibilities for dependents, and limited funds.

A woman undergoing an abortion understands all too well the reproductive consequences of unprotected sex and is often ashamed and guilty. She may insist that she will never let this happen again. She needs empathic counseling so that she can acknowledge and address any problems that made her vulnerable to the problem pregnancy.

The Client's Emotional Reactions

A woman's logical analysis of her situation can't be separated from her feelings. Having a child or not having one is never only a rational matter, or even mostly so. Though the thinking and the feeling are inseparable, they are separated here for purposes of discussion. Nothing in this section should be taken to mean that a woman is "too emotional" to make a decision about her own pregnancy.

Normal Reactions

Normal emotional reactions to a problem pregnancy and a contemplated abortion are very variable. There are also individual and cultural differences in clients' willingness and abilities to reveal intimate emotions to a stranger and in their openness to counseling as a process. Neither a flood of tears nor a carefully controlled demeanor is a sign of an underlying emotional problem. Some women may act totally unconcerned; this may indicate an unwillingness to engage with the counselor or difficulty dealing with the emotional implications of abortion. The progress of the interview will help the counselor to distinguish between these two possibilities.

The client may need help accepting her own feelings. She may feel rage at the man with whom she created the pregnancy or at family members who are not offering the help she needs, guilt over the affair or the unintended conception, anxiety over the consequences of her choices, sadness over the impending loss of the pregnancy, or relief at the thought that the pregnancy will soon be over. These feelings may coexist or alternate. It may be difficult for her friends and family to keep up with and respond to them.

Focusing on the Decision

The time frame for decisions about a pregnancy does not allow for the complete exploration and working through of conflicting emotions and painful relationships. The counselor can help a client to identify issues that may deserve attention after the immediate crisis is resolved. It can be difficult to assess the significance of problems because the crisis can amplify the client's perceptions and feelings. When the client has decided what to do and has done it, she will focus her attention either on preparing for the birth of her child or on resuming the pattern of her life before the pregnancy.

It is possible, and common, to know that abortion is the right decision and yet to feel terribly sad about the circumstances and the possibility of a new life lost. The counselor needs to prepare the client and her significant others for a wide variety of emotional responses after an abortion. The most common predominant emotion is relief, but some women also experience transient guilt and sadness.

Distinguishing Strong Feelings From Psychological Problems: The Why and How of Referral

There is no evidence that abortion causes psychiatric illness. Psychiatric illness does occur in the context of abortion, but less frequently than in the context of childbirth. Occasionally the reactions and behaviors of a client are too demanding for the context of counseling and require formal clinical evaluation.

Signs and symptoms indicating a need for diagnosis and treatment include the following:

- An inability to make up her mind about what to do, even with the support and structure of counseling
- Progressively deteriorating function

- Worsening interference with sleep, appetite, concentration, and/or energy
- Significant deleterious effects on otherwise positive relationships with significant others
- Abuse of alcohol or other substances
- Engaging in behavior potentially dangerous to herself or others, such as reckless driving or spending time in the company of persons known to be violent
- Serious thoughts about suicide
- Overwhelming sadness or guilt
- Bizarre experiences or thoughts, such as hallucinations, delusions, or paranoia. Paranoia consists of a belief, without foundation in reality, that others actively intend to harm the client. This must be distinguished from suspiciousness or a general sense of injustice.

Suicidal ideation should prompt immediate evaluation by a psychiatrist—err on the side of safety. The patient should not be left alone, even for a moment. Symptoms of psychosis and clinical depression are also best handled by a psychiatrist; they may necessitate the use of medication and/or hospitalization. Just as the clinic will have medical backup for emergencies, the counselor may want to arrange in advance for the possibility of a psychiatric emergency. This can be done either by establishing a working relationship with a local psychiatrist or by locating a nearby hospital emergency department. These events are very rare, but it is best to be prepared.

Because psychiatric illness and care are still stigmatized in our society, a counselor may feel awkward about suggesting a mental health referral for a client. The client may not recognize that she has a problem; she may be talking to the counselor only because it is required before obtaining an abortion. Or she may realize that she has a problem but attribute it to others or to external circumstances rather than to psychiatric illness or inner conflict. The counselor may fear that the client will interpret the referral as a statement that she is "crazy."

A referral will make more sense to a client if it is explained in terms of her own symptoms, by saying, for example, "I'm concerned about the difficulty you're having sleeping," or "I'm not having success in helping you decide what to do; I would like you to consult with an expert." It's an advantage when the expert is someone with whom the counselor works on a regular basis and who is particularly knowledgeable about this type of situation.

It may also happen that the experience of the problem pregnancy and the usefulness of counseling sensitizes the client to unresolved psychological problems and prompts her to request a referral for further psychotherapeutic work. The counselor can undertake that work or can refer the patient to a local practitioner.

Decisions in the Context of Psychiatric Illness and Treatment

It may also happen that a woman in ongoing therapy with a clinical professional experiences a problem pregnancy. An abortion counselor or a mental health professional with a particular interest in the psychological aspects of women's reproductive health may be of help. Psychiatric illness, even when it is severe, is not a criterion for depriving a woman of her right to choose or for mandating an abortion. Psychiatric illness may be an important factor in a woman's reproductive decision; it may cause her to lose custody of her children, trigger recurrent postpartum depression, or make it difficult to care for her children. A woman must have access to the full range of legal reproductive health services, including abortion, even if she is psychiatrically hospitalized. In those extremely rare cases in which she cannot comprehend the decision because of mental disability, a guardian should be appointed to decide in her best interest.

Sometimes an abortion decision arises when a patient has taken psychoactive or other medication in the first weeks before pregnancy was diagnosed. Very little is known about the effects of most medications on the embryo and fetus. The patient or the doctor who prescribed the medication may wish to confer with a subspecialist in this area in order to bring as much information as possible to the decision about the pregnancy. A great deal depends upon the nature of the medication; there is often no cause for alarm, but the client always deserves all the scientific information that is currently available.

Problem pregnancies also occur in the course of treatment for a milder mental illness. The information in this book may be useful to patient and therapist alike by helping them to understand the historical and legal context of abortion, the procedures used, and the process of locating an abortion provider. The therapist, like the abortion counselor, can assist a woman in thinking through her values, feelings, circumstances, and plans so that she can make an autonomous, informed, and considered choice. Although the therapist may prefer one choice or the other and may share that perspective with the patient if asked, the therapist must be careful not to insinuate that preference into the therapeutic work.

Difficult Patients

Some people are very difficult to deal with. Generally the difficulty derives from personality style. Counselors also have to know themselves. A particular patient may be irksome, enraging, or depressing, not because of the client's behavior, but because, or partly because, she reminds the counselor of one or more people in the counselor's own life. This can happen regularly with a certain kind of client or out of the blue when a client has some specific, perhaps minor, trait that evokes a painful situation in the life of the counselor. A counselor may be vulnerable because of an ongoing difficulty in her current life, such as a rebellious adolescent child, a troubled love affair, or an ill relative.

Some such experiences are inevitable in the professional life of a counselor. It is essential to accept that fact and to learn to recognize the potential impact on the counseling process. Usually these situations can be resolved with a little reflection. If the problem persists and interferes with counseling, the counselor will want to confer with a supervisor, colleague, or other mental health professional.

Most of the time, clients who seem irritating would seem so to anyone. People's personality styles feel natural and inevitable to themselves. Their styles give them trouble only when they provoke opposition, avoidance, or hostility in others. When that happens, the person with the difficult personality attributes the trouble to the other person and not to herself, saying things such as "Other people won't give me the help I need," "Other people are messy," or "Other people don't realize how bad I feel."

It is sometimes reassuring when exasperated by a challenging client to remember that the client's annoying behavior is probably related to her anxiety. Some personality styles are so chronically exaggerated as to constitute personality disorders. It is useful to recognize the specific constellations of troublesome behaviors, both because this recognition will offer the counselor a helpful sense of objectivity and because the counselor can then approach the client in a specifically helpful way. The counselor must take care not to label the client with a diagnosis in a demeaning or stigmatizing way.

Following are descriptions of some problematic personality styles and suggestions for coping with them. Not uncommonly, one person has a mixture of several.

- Dependent: A dependent person hangs on the counselor's every word and constantly clings to others for direction and support. She feels that she cannot make decisions or act on them on her own. The counselor will have to make it clear just what she can and cannot offer the patient and firmly express her conviction that the patient must, can, and will make her own decision.
- Histrionic: The histrionic person, afraid of being ignored, invests every event and feeling with high drama. The counselor must avoid getting caught up in the intensity of such a client's emotion and help the client to get down to the realities of her situation.
- Narcissistic: A narcissistic person, feeling inferior on the inside, acts superior on the outside. She acts entitled to extra attention, extra time, and extra services. The counselor should carefully spell out the services offered to everyone and then give neither more nor less to this type of client.
- Borderline: The client with a borderline personality disorder is often hostile. She tends to see things in black and white, so that some people seem angelic and most people seem mean and withholding. Often her views toward the same individual alternate between these poles according to her most recent experience. Her relationships are therefore unstable and intense. Dealing with a person with a border-

line personality disorder is like weathering a storm; keep your bearings and hold on tight! These clients make you angry, because they are angry. Inside, they experience considerable, constant pain. They engage in impulsive and self-destructive behaviors. In response to the crisis of a problem pregnancy, however, they can sometimes produce focused and effective responses.

- Obsessive-Compulsive: An obsessive-compulsive individual is oriented to data, schedules, and details. She may bring written lists of questions and symptoms. Rather than trying to get such a client to "loosen up" her whole personality in the middle of a life crisis, the counselor can put the client's style to use. Give her as much printed information as possible, have her prioritize her question list, let her keep charts and journals, and put directions and procedures in writing for her.

Clients With Genetic and Medical Indications for Abortion

Women who must consider abortion because of defects found in the fetus or because their own health makes pregnancy and childbirth too risky have special feelings and needs related to those circumstances, in addition to whatever other problems their lives entail.[2] The pregnancy may have been much desired by such a client. Specialized medical information will have to be provided by experts in genetics or in whatever medical condition the woman has. She will want to know not only the risks in this pregnancy but also her reproductive prospects for the future.

These women often feel that their own bodies have failed. The prospect of ending the pregnancy may represent a disappointment to the man involved, even a loss of their only opportunity to have a child together. Tensions over the reproductive problem may severely strain the relationship. The couple, and even their families, may exchange accusations about the source of the defect or illness and the desirability of the couple's relationship. The woman who is medically ill feels the inability to bear a child as another assault on her participation in the ordinary joys and prospects of life. If she is not involved in a committed relationship, she may have especially hoped for a child to love and be loved by, to be her family.

These clients are at increased risk for depression after abortion. Though the depression is perfectly understandable, it should not be ignored. The client, counselor, and other health care providers should be alert for persistent (lasting more than 2 weeks) depressed mood; crying spells; decreases in appetite, sleep, concentration, and ability to enjoy people and activities; and preoccupation with guilt, death, and even suicide. Depression is a painful and debilitating illness that can be effectively treated with antidepressants and/or psychotherapy.

These clients are likely to provoke strong feelings in the counselor as well. Regardless of the genetic or medical diagnosis, the counselor cannot assume that the client will either continue or end the pregnancy. Some women's personal or religious convictions ultimately require them to bear any child they conceive. Some women will risk their health and even their lives to bear a child. Others prefer to abort if there is any suspicion of defect or illness, no matter how slight. Their choices must be respected.

In Closing

The ideas outlined in this chapter represent ideals. Abortion counselors operate under severe time constraints, helping women in difficult, sometimes tragic, circumstances to make and carry out painful decisions. Their clients may be anywhere from the beginning to the end of their reproductive life spans, rich or poor, well acclimated or newly arrived, pampered or abused. They may be hungry for counseling services that are not available or resentful of the counseling they are required to undergo.

Counselors are often confronted with abortion service limitations beyond their control and sometimes confronted by threatening demonstrators. They cannot guarantee their clients an outcome that is "right" or happy. For many women, the counselor is the only person who listens with concern and impartiality.

Counseling can be the cornerstone of the autonomous and informed decision making that is associated with the optimal outcome of reproductive decisions. Counselors therefore make a valuable and generous contribution to the health of our society.

Resource Directory

Abortion

General Information

The following are sources of up-to-date statistics and other general information about abortion and abortion providers, as well as further resources and assistance.

Alan Guttmacher Institute
120 Wall Street
New York, NY 10005
Telephone: (212) 248-1111
Fax: 212.248.1951
E-mail: info@agi-usa.org
World Wide Web:
   http://www.agi-usa.org

The Alan Guttmacher Institute provides the latest in abortion research, facts, and figures, in addition to information about teenage sexuality and pregnancy.

American Civil Liberties Union
Reproductive Freedom Project
125 Broad Street, 18th Floor
New York, NY 10004
Telephone: (212) 549-2500

Women's Health Rights Coalition
558 Capp Street
San Francisco, CA 94110
Telephone: (415) 647-2697

The Women's Health Rights Coalition publishes a newsletter and fact sheets about abortion and other women's health topics.

Feminist Women's Health Centers
3401 Folsom Boulevard, Suite A
Sacramento, CA 95816
Telephone: (916) 451-0621

National Abortion Federation
1775 Massachusetts Avenue NW, Suite 600
Washington, DC 20036
Telephone: (202) 667-5881
Hotline: (800) 772-9100
Fax: 202.667.5890

You can call this hotline to check the credentials of any abortion provider or other agency.

National Abortion and Reproductive Rights Action
League (NARAL)
1156 15th Street NW
Washington, DC 20005
Telephone: (202) 973-3000
Legal Library telephone: (202) 973-3018
Fax: 202.973.3099

National Organization for Women
1000 16th Street NW, Suite 700
Washington, DC 20036
Telephone: (202) 331-0066
Fax: 202.785.8576
E-mail: now@now.org
World Wide Web:
  http://www.now.org

 National Women's Health Network
514 10th Street NW
Washington, DC 20004
Telephone: (202) 347-1140
Fax: 202.347.1168

Pro-Choice Resource Center
174 East Boston Post Road
Mamaroneck, NY 10543
Telephone: (914) 381-3792

The Pro-Choice Resource Center provides instruction and assistance for pro-choice grassroots groups.

Reproductive Health Technologies Project
1818 N Street NW, Suite 450
Washington, DC 20036
Telephone: (202) 530-2900
Fax: 202.530.2901

The Reproductive Health Technologies Project provides information on the latest in abortion procedure technology, including RU-486.

Financial Assistance

Hershey Abortion Assistance Fund
c/o Pro-Choice Resources
3255 Hennepin Avenue S, #255
Minneapolis, MN 55408
Telephone: (612) 825-2000

The Hershey Abortion Assistance Fund provides referrals and financial assistance for abortion. Callers may call collect.

National Network of Abortion Funds
c/o Civil Liberties and Public Policy Programs
Hampshire College
Amherst, MA 01002
Telephone: (413) 582-5645
Fax: 413.582-5620
E-mail: clpp@hamp.hampshire.edu
World Wide Web:
   http://hamp.hampshire.edu/~clpp/nnaf

NNAF provides support and technical assistance to local abortion funds across the country, encourages and enables the creation of new abortion funds in areas where they do not exist, engages in coalition work on the national level on issues of access to abortion with special emphasis on funding, and provides visibility and a voice for women currently being denied their right to a safe, legal abortion.

Planned Parenthood Federation of America, Inc.
810 Seventh Avenue
New York, NY 10019
Telephone: (212) 541-7800
E-mail: communications@ppfa.org
World Wide Web:
   http://www.ppfa.org/ppfa

Planned Parenthood arranges reduced or deferred payment for women in need.

Informative Reading Material

American College of Obstetricians and Gynecologists
409 12th Street SW
Washington, DC 20024-2188
Resource Center telephone: (202) 863-2518
Fax: 202.484.5107
World Wide Web:
  http://www.acog.com

A pamphlet from ACOG entitled "Important Medical Facts About Induced Abortion" is available in single copies or in bulk quantities.

Bonavoglia A (ed): *The Choices We Made*. New York,
Random House, 1991

This is a book of women's stories, told in their own words, about their experiences with abortion. It should be available at your local bookstore or library.

Boston Women's Health Book Collective: *The New Our*
***Bodies, Ourselves*. New York, Touchstone, 1992**

This book, written by and for women, contains chapters on birth control, pregnancy decisions, abortion, pregnancy, childbirth, violence against women, and many other highly relevant topics. It should be available at your local bookstore or library.

Weddington S: A Question of Choice. New York, Penguin, 1993

This is a book by the attorney who argued and won the landmark 1973 *Roe v. Wade* abortion rights case before the Supreme Court of the United States. It gives the reader insight into the circumstances that led to that case and the legal, philosophical, and personal reasoning that went into it.

Legal Information

The Center for Reproductive Law and Policy
120 Wall Street, 18th floor
New York, NY 10005
Telephone: (212) 514-5534
Fax: 212.514.5538

The Center for Reproductive Law and Policy provides up-to-the-minute information about national and local laws and law enforcement concerning abortion.

Pro-Choice Religious Organizations

Catholics for a Free Choice
1436 U Street NW, Suite 301
Washington, DC 20009
Telephone: (202) 986-6093
Fax: 202.332.7995
e-mail: cfc@igc.atc.org
World Wide Web:
    http://www.igc.org/catholicvote

Religious Coalition for Reproductive Choice
1025 Vermont Avenue NW, Suite 1130
Washington, DC 20005
Telephone: (202) 628-7700
Fax: 202.628.7716
E-mail: inforcrc.org
World Wide Web:
   http://www.rcrc.org

The Religious Coalition for Reproductive Choice is a coalition whose membership represents several Protestant Christian denominations, Jewish groups, and other religiously affiliated organizations.

Racial and Ethnic Group Organizations

Asian and Pacific Islanders for Reproductive Health
310 8th Street, Suite 100
Oakland, CA 94607
Telephone: (510) 268-8988
Fax: 510.268.8181
E-mail: apirh@igc.org

National Latina Health Organization
PO Box 7567
Oakland, CA 94601
Telephone: (510) 534-1362
Fax: 510. 534.1364
E-mail: latinahlth@aol.com

Native American Women's Health Education Resource Center
PO Box 572
Lake Andes, SD 57356
Telephone: (605) 487-7072
Fax: 605.487.7964

Adoption

Adoption Crossroads
356 East 74th Street, Suite 2
New York, NY 10021
Telephone: (212) 988-0110
Fax: 212.988.0291
E-mail: cera@idt.net
World Wide Web:
    http://www.adoptioncrossroads.org

American Adoption Congress
1000 Connecticut Avenue NW, Suite 9
Washington, DC 20036
Telephone: (202) 483-3399

National Adoption Information Clearinghouse
1400 I Street NW, Suite 1275
Washington, DC 20005

National Council for Adoption
1930 17th Street NW
Washington, DC 20009-6207
Telephone: (202) 328-1200
Fax: 202.332.0935
E-mail: NCFA@Juno.com
World Wide Web:
    http://www.ncfa-usa.org

Domestic Violence

National Domestic Violence Hotlines

(800) 799-SAFE (799-7233)
TDD for the hearing impaired: (800) 787-3224

Established as part of the 1994 Violence Against Women Act, the hotline provides help for victims of domestic violence across the country 24 hours a day, 7 days a week, 365 days a year. The service is toll free and operates throughout the United States, Puerto Rico, and the Virgin Islands.

Books

Davidson S, NiCarthy G: *You Can Be Free: An Easy-to-Read Handbook for Abused Women*. Seattle, WA: Seal Press, 1989

DeFrain J: *On Our Own: A Single Parent's Survival Guide*. Lexington, MA, Lexington Books, 1987

Mental Health

American Psychiatric Association
APA Department MH
1400 K Street NW, Suite 501
Washington, DC 20005
Telephone: (202) 682-6220

American Psychological Association
750 First Street NE
Washington, DC 20002
Telephone: (202) 336-6080 (local)
or
(800) 950-2000
Fax: 202.336.6069
World Wide Web:
   http://www.apa.org

National Alliance for the Mentally Ill
200 North Glebe Road, Suite 1015
Arlington, VA 22203-3754
Telephone: (703) 524-7600 (local)
or
(800) 950-6264 (help line)
Fax: 703.524.9094
E-mail: namioffc@nami.org
World Wide Web:
   http://www.nami.org

National Depressive and Manic-Depressive Association
730 North Franklin Street, Suite 501
Chicago, IL 60610
Telephone: (312) 642-0049(local)
or
(800) 82-NDMDA (826-3632)
Fax: 312.642-7243
World Wide Web:
   http://www.ndmda.org

National Institute of Mental Health
Public Inquiries, Room 7C-02
5600 Fishers Lane
Rockville, MD 20857
Telephone: (800) 421-4211 (Depression Hotline)
Fax: 301.443.2578
World Wide Web:
  http://www.nimh.nih.gov

National Mental Health Association Information Center
1021 Prince Street
Alexandria, VA 22314
Telephone: (703) 684-7722 (local)
or
(800) 969-NMHA (969-6642)
Fax: 703.684.5968

References

Chapter 1

1. Adler NE, David HP, Major BN, et al: "Psychological Responses After Abortion." *Science* 248(4951):41–44, 1990
2. Koonin LM, Smith JC, Ramick M: "Abortion Surveillance—United States, 1990." *Morbidity and Mortality Weekly Report CDC Surveillance Summary (NE9)* 42(SS-6):29–57, 1993
3. Forrest JD: "Unintended Pregnancy Among American Women." *Family Planning Perspectives* 19:76, 1987
4. Gold RB: *Abortion and Women's Health: A Turning Point for America?* New York, Alan Guttmacher Institute, 1990
5. Schusterman LR: "The Psychosocial Factors of the Abortion Experience: A Critical Review." *Psychology of Women Quarterly* 1:79–102, 1976
6. Adler NE, David HP, Major BN, et al: "Psychological Factors in Abortion: A Review." *American Psychologist* 47(10):1194–1204, 1992
7. Adler NE, David HP, Major BN, et al: "Psychological Responses After Abortion." *Science* 248(4951):41–44, 1990
8. American Medical Association Council on Scientific Affairs: "Induced Termination of Pregnancy Before and After Roe v Wade: Trends in the Mortality and Morbidity of Women." *Journal of the American Medical Association* 268(22):3231–3239, 1992
9. Grimes DA: "The Morbidity and Mortality of Pregnancy: Still Risky Business." *American Journal of Obstetrics and Gynecology* 170(5 pt 2):1489–1494, 1994

Chapter 2

1. Tribe LH: *Abortion: The Clash of Absolutes*. New York, WW Norton, 1990
2. Bonavoglia A (ed): *The Choices We Made*. New York, Random House, 1991
3. Devereux G: *A Study of Abortion in Primitive Societies, Revised Edition*. New York, International Universities Press, 1976
4. Savage M: "The Law of Abortion in the Union of Soviet Socialist Republics and the People's Republic of China: Women's Rights in Two Socialist Countries." *Stanford Law Review* 40:250–271, 1988
5. Peipert JF, Domagalski L, Boardman L, et al: "College Women and Contraceptive Use, 1975–1995." *New England Journal of Medicine* 335(3):211, 1996
6. Henshaw SK, Kost K: "Abortion Patients in 1994-1995: Characteristics and Contraceptive Use." *Family Planning Perspectives* 28(4):140–147, 158, 1996
7. Henshaw SK, Silverman J: "The Characteristics and Prior Contraceptive Use of U.S. Abortion Patients." *Family Planning Perspectives* 20(4):158–168, 1988
8. Terrell J, Modell M: "Anthropology and Adoption." *American Anthropologist* 96(1):155–161, 1994

Chapter 3

1. Cates W Jr, Rochat RW: "Illegal abortions in the United States: 1972–1974." *Family Planning Perspectives* 8:86–92, 1976
2. Tietz C, Henshaw SK: *Induced Abortion: A World Review*. New York, Alan Guttmacher Institute, 1986
3. Alan Guttmacher Institute: "Abortion in the U.S.: Two Centuries of Experience." *Issues in Brief* 2(4):1–4, 1982
4. National Abortion Federation: *Fact Sheet: Safety of Abortion*. Washington, DC, National Abortion Federation, 1992
5. American Medical Association Council on Scientific Affairs: "Induced Termination of Pregnancy Before and After Roe V Wade: Trends in the Mortality and Morbidity of Women." *Journal of the American Medical Association* 268(22):3231–3239, 1992
6. Grimes DA: "The Morbidity and Mortality of Pregnancy: Still Risky Business." *Am J Obstet Gynecol* 170(5 pt 2):1489–1494, 1994

7. David HP: "Induced Abortion: Psychosocial Aspects," in *Gynecology and Obstetrics*. Edited by Sciama JJ. Philadelphia, PA, Harper & Row, 1995

8. Henshaw SK, Van Vort J: "Abortion services in the United States, 1991 and 1992." *Family Planning Perspectives* 26(3):100–106, 112, 1994

9. Koonin LM, Smith JC, Ramick M: "Abortion surveillance—United States, 1990." *Morbidity and Mortality Weekly Report CDC Surveillance Summary* 42(SS-6):29–57, 1993

10. Forrest JD: "Unintended Pregnancy Among American Women." *Family Planning Perspectives* 19:76–79, 1987

11. Gold RB: *Abortion and Women's Health: A Turning Point for America?* New York, Alan Guttmacher Institute, 1990

12. Henshaw SK, Kost K: "Abortion Patients in 1994–1995: Characteristics and Contraceptive Use." *Family Planning Perspectives* 28(4):140–147, 1996

13. Lindsay J, Manserrat C: *Adoption Awareness: A Guide for Teachers, Counselors, Nurses, and Caring Others*. Buena Park, CA, Morning Glory Press, 1989

14. Flango VE, Flango CR: "How Many Children Were Adopted in 1992." *Child Welfare* 74(5):1018–1032, 1995

15. Genevie L, Margolies E: *The Motherhood Report*. New York, Macmillan, 1987

16. Chilman CS: *Adolescent Sexuality in a Changing American Society*. New York, Wiley-Interscience, 1983

17. Mott FL, Marsiglio W: "Early Childbearing and the Completion of High School." *Family Planning Perspectives* 17:234–237, 1985

18. Alan Guttmacher Institute: *Sex and America's Teenagers*. New York, Alan Guttmacher Institute, 1994

19. David HP, Dytrych Z, Matejcek Z, et al (eds): *Born Unwanted: Developmental Effects of Denied Abortion*. New York, Springer, 1988

20. Forssman H, Thuwe I: "Continued Follow-Up Study of 120 Persons Born After Refusal of Application for Therapeutic Abortion." *Acta Psychiatrica Scandinavica* 64:142–146, 1981

Chapter 4

1. Henshaw SK, Kost K: "Parental Involvement in Minors' Abortion Decisions." *Family Planning Perspectives* 24(5):196–207, 213, 1992

2. Alan Guttmacher Institute: *Sex and America's Teenagers*. New York, Alan Guttmacher Institute, 1994

3. Torres A, Forrest JD: "Why Do Women Have Abortions?" *Family Planning Perspectives* 20:158, 1988
4. Henshaw SK, Van Vort J: "Abortion services in the United States, 1991 and 1992." *Family Planning Perspectives* 26(3):100–106, 112, 1994
5. Tough P: "Forum: Davenport, Abortion, and Common Ground." *Harper's Magazine,* August 1996, pp 39–49
6. Evans MI, Gleicher E, Feingold E, et al: "The Fiscal Impact of the Medicaid Abortion Funding Ban in Michigan." *Obstetrics and Gynecology* 82(4):555–560, 1993

Chapter 5

1. Stubblefield PG: "Induced Abortion: Indications, Counseling, and Services," in *Gynecology and Obstetrics.* Edited by Sciama JJ. Philadelphia, PA, Harper & Row, 1995
2. Gold RB: *Abortion and Women's Health: A Turning Point for America?* New York, Alan Guttmacher Institute, 1990
3. Henshaw SK: "Induced Abortion: Epidemiological Aspects," in *Gynecology and Obstetrics.* Edited by Sciama JJ. Philadelphia, PA, Harper & Row, 1995
4. Lawson HW, Atrash HK, Saftlas AF, et al: "Abortion surveillance: United States, 1984–1985." *Morbidity and Mortality Weekly Report CDC Surveillance Summary* 38(55-2):11–45, 1989
5. Stubblefield PG: "Surgical Techniques for First Trimester Abortion," in *Gynecology and Obstetrics.* Edited by Sciama JJ. Philadelphia, PA, Harper & Row, 1995
6. Nichols KA: "Elective abortion," in *Textbook of Women's Health.* Edited by Wallis LA. Boston, MA, Little, Brown, in press
7. Stika CS: "Antiprogestins," in *Gynecology and Obstetrics.* Edited by Sciama JJ. Philadelphia, PA, Harper & Row, 1995
8. Alan Guttmacher Institute: *Abortion in the United States: Facts in Brief.* New York, Alan Guttmacher Institute, 1995
9. Tarani A, Lavechia C, Franceschi S, et al: "Abortion and Breast-Cancer Risk." *International Journal of Cancer* 65(4):401–405, 1996

Chapter 6

1. Bonavoglia A (ed): *The Choices We Made.* New York, Random House, 1991

2. Segers MC: "The Loyal Opposition: Catholics for a Free Choice," in *The Catholic Church and the Politics of Abortion*. Edited by Byrnes TA, Segers MC. Boulder, CO, Westview Press, 1992, pp 169–184

3. Feldman P: "Sexuality, Birth Control, and Childbirth in Orthodox Jewish Tradition." *Canadian Medical Association Journal* 146(1):29–33, 1992

4. Tribe LH: *Abortion: The Clash of Absolutes*. New York, WW Norton, 1990

5. Rosenblatt R: "A History of Contradiction," in *Life Itself: Abortion in the American Mind*. Edited by Rosenblatt R. New York, Vintage Books, 1992, pp 49–98

6. Sachdev P: *International Handbook on Abortion*. New York, Greenwood Press, 1988

7. Cook EA, Jelen TG, Wilcox C: "Measuring Public Attitudes on Abortion: Methodological and Substantive Considerations." *Family Planning Perspectives* 25(3):118–121, 145, 1993

8. Rosenblatt R: "A Note on Opinion Polls," in *Life Itself: Abortion in the American Mind*. Edited by Rosenblatt R. New York, Vintage Books, 1992, pp 185–189

9. Tenvergert E, Gillespie MW, Kingma J, Klasen H: "Abortion Attitudes, 1984–1987–1988: Effects of Item Order and Dimensionality." *Perceptual and Motor Skills* 72(2):627–642, 1992

Chapter 7

1. Barnett ER, Pittman CB, Ragan CK, et al: *Family Violence: Interaction Strategies*. Publ No DHHS (OHDS) 80-30258. Washington, DC, U.S. Government Printing Office, 1980

2. Mertus JA: "Fake Abortion Clinics: The Threat to Reproductive Self-Determination." *Women and Health* 16(1):95–113, 1990

Chapter 9

1. Stotland NL: "The Myth of the Abortion Trauma Syndrome." *Journal of the American Medical Association* 268:2078–2079, 1992

2. Aarons ZA: "Therapeutic Abortion and the Psychiatrist," in *Scientific Proceedings of the 123rd Annual Meeting of the American Psychiatric Association*. Washington, DC, American Psychiatric Association, 1967, pp 163–164

3. Brown SS, Eisenberg L (eds): *The Best Intentions: Unintended Pregnancy and the Well-Being of Children and Families.* Washington, DC, National Academy Press, 1995
4. Depression Guideline Panel: *Depression in Primary Care, Vol 1: Detection and Diagnosis. Clinical Practice Guideline No 5.* AHCPR Publication No. 93-0550. Rockville, MD, U.S. Department of Health and Human Services, Public Health Service Agency for Health Care Policy and Research, 1993
5. American Psychiatric Association: *Diagnostic and Statistical Manual of Mental Disorders, 4th Edition.* Washington, DC, American Psychiatric Association, 1994
6. Cassem NH: "Depression," in *Massachusetts General Hospital Handbook of General Hospital Psychiatry.* Edited by Cassem NH. St. Louis, MO, CV Mosby, 1991, pp 237–268

Chapter 11

1. Kiernan KE: "Teenage Marriage and Marital Breakdown: A Longitudinal Study." *Population Studies* 40(1):35–54, 1986
2. Henshaw SK, Kost K: "Parental Involvement in Minors' Abortion Decisions. *Family Planning Perspectives* 24(5):196–207, 213, 1992

Chapter 12

1. American Medical Association Council on Scientific Affairs: "Adolescents as Victims of Family Violence." *Journal of the American Medical Association* 270(15):1850–1856, 1993
2. Kolker A, Burke BM: "Grieving the Wanted Child: Ramifications of Abortion After Prenatal Diagnosis of Abnormality." Health Care for Women International 14(6):513–526, 1993

Index

Page numbers in **bold** type refer to tables or figures.